Essential
Oils
H A N D B O O K

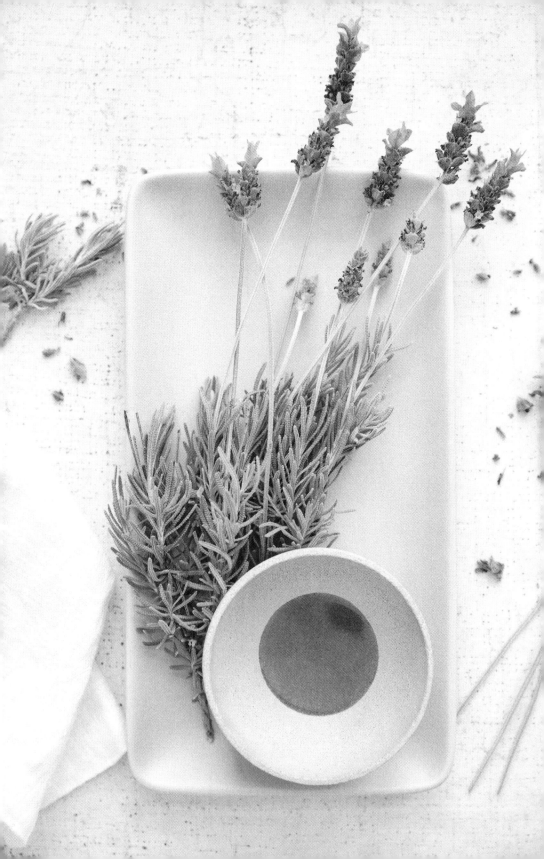

Recipes for Natural Living

Essential Oils

HANDBOOK

AMY LEIGH MERCREE

Foreword by STACY ROMILLAH, *Certifed Aromatherapist*

STERLING
New York

STERLING
New York

An Imprint of Sterling Publishing Co., Inc.
1166 Avenue of the Americas
New York, NY 10036

ISBN 978-1-4549-2898-0

Distributed in Canada by Sterling Publishing Co., Inc.
c/o Canadian Manda Group, 664 Annette Street
Toronto, Ontario M6S 2C8, Canada
Distributed in the United Kingdom by GMC Distribution Services
Castle Place, 166 High Street, Lewes, East Sussex BN7 1XU, England
Distributed in Australia by NewSouth Books
45 Beach Street, Coogee, NSW 2034, Australia

For information about custom editions, special sales, and premium and corporate purchases,
please contact Sterling Special Sales at 800-805-5489 or specialsales@sterlingpublishing.com.

Manufactured in the United States of America

2 4 6 8 10 9 7 5 3 1

sterlingpublishing.com

Interior design by Christine Heun
Cover design by Elizabeth Lindy

For Picture Credits, see page 220

CONTENTS

FOREWORD

Modern aromatherapy, the "medicine of the future," draws its wisdom from experiences that are rooted deep in antiquity. Since the times of ancient Egypt, across the continents and millennia to the foundations of Chinese medicine, essential oils have held a central place in health, culture, and beauty.

Myrrh was once valued even more than gold. Mary Magdalene anointed the feet of Jesus with Spikenard oil, a gift of kings. Frankincense was mixed with charcoal to make classic black eyeliner for Egyptians of old. Now, for the first time in world history, we have easy access to the oils once reserved only for royalty, or at least the very wealthy.

Essential oils are a potent distillation of the non–water-soluble essence of plants. They are so concentrated that it takes over 130 pounds of rose petals to make a single ounce of Rose oil. One drop of Peppermint essential oil is equivalent to drinking 30 cups of strong peppermint tea. If you want to boost your physical, emotional, or spiritual well-being quickly, and in a big way, aromatherapy is your new best friend.

We are living at a time when, more than ever, we need the knowledge and skills to take care of ourselves. We are exposed to levels of chemicals, stress, and pollution that strain our immune systems and speed aging. Since we are living longer, we need new tools to help us experience a high quality of life, vitality, and youthfulness into our later decades. This is easy to do if we start early and incorporate the gifts of the emerging science of wellness, of which aromatherapy is central.

Essential oils are a superpower from the plant world. They enhance your well-being, don't require a prescription, are easily accessible, and can support every aspect of your health and beauty.

The first time I heard about essential oils, I was on a commercial fishing boat in the Bering Sea off the coast of Alaska, reading a massage magazine.

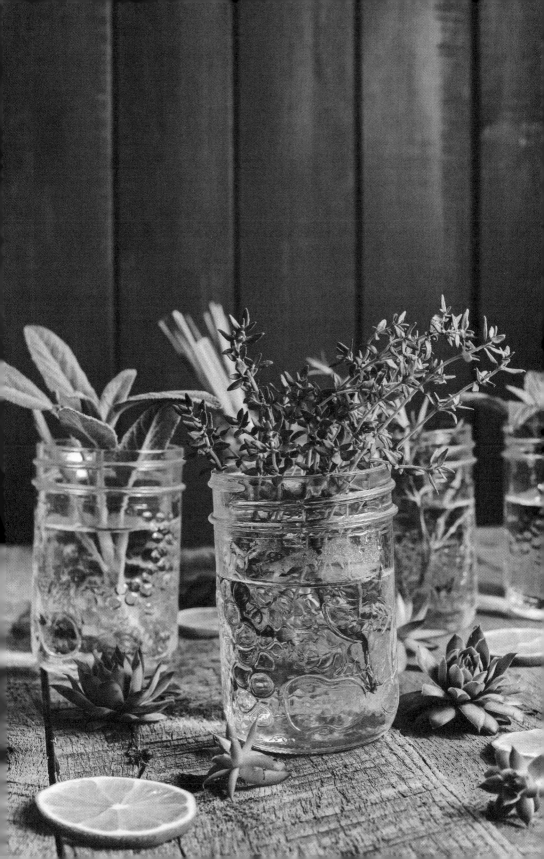

An article about essential oils captured my bioscience-obsessed mind and spurred me to order every oil from the ad I saw on the next page. Next, I ordered every book I could find that was written in English. The year was 1989.

Fast-forward nearly 30 years and you have hundreds of essential oil companies to order from, heaps of scientific evidence to substantiate the efficacy of the oils at your fingertips, and millions of Google search results.

Since 1989, I've used essential oils to support hundreds of patients in my medical practice, flavor my meals, bless ceremonies, anoint my body with heavenly fragrance, clean my kitchen and bathroom, replace chemical-laden body care products, fill my home with mood-lifting scents, and treat every health challenge my family has faced.

Aromatherapy is also a key aspect of my meditation practice and the guided inner journeys I lead people on. They can help one feel centered and grounded, balanced, and calm. There are reasons that spiritual practitioners the world over incorporate incense in their work. Essential oils help us release our monkey-mind focus on the mundane and open us to experiences of a divine nature.

Essential oils have been used in Asian medicine for thousands of years, but because of locally limited growing climates, processing abilities, and trade routes, essential oils were largely unavailable or unaffordable to the general population. If the vast majority of Asians had access to oils the way we now do, Asian medicine, Ayurvedic medicine, and herbalism around the world would be focused on essential oils. It just wasn't possible before now!

As an acupuncturist, I use essential oils to create herbal formulas that support my clients' well-being. Oftentimes, I find essential oils more effective than the herbal tea or pill formulas of Asian medicine.

They are always part of my cancer-prevention regimen. They provide detoxification support, help people overcome digestive challenges, balance hormones, alleviate the symptoms of menopause, increase brain functioning, decrease inflammation and pain from injury and disease, relieve tension, and clear headaches. The list goes on and on. I use them with nearly every client.

Personally, *I always* have essential oils with me. I feel more confident to be able to address anything that comes my way when I have the power of an extensive herbal apothecary contained in a small bag of oils that fits in my purse.

I have this confidence because I use high-quality medicinal oils. When it comes to aromatherapy, quality matters. Just as you would not take any white pill and hope it would work like a prescription, you cannot use any scented oil and hope it will support your health. Nothing Amy shares with you in this book will matter if you aren't using pure oils.

I recommend doing your due diligence and choosing a company that publishes the chemical analyses of its products. All companies will say their oils are pure and natural, but it's up to you to research each company and find the highest-quality oils you can. (Hint: Ordering directly from individual companies online is your best bet!)

With Amy's experienced guidance, a world of empowered wellness is about to open up to you! I hope it blesses your life, as it does mine.

STACY ROMILLAH *is an internationallly certifed Aromatherapist and has a Master's of Acupuncture.*

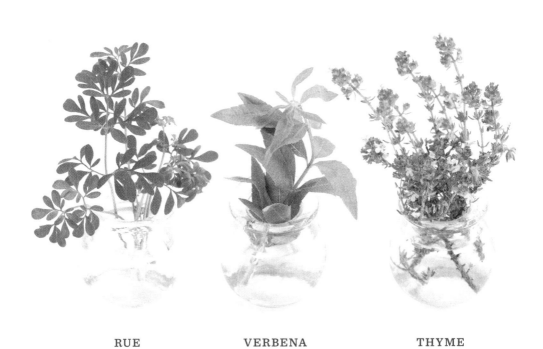

RUE   VERBENA   THYME

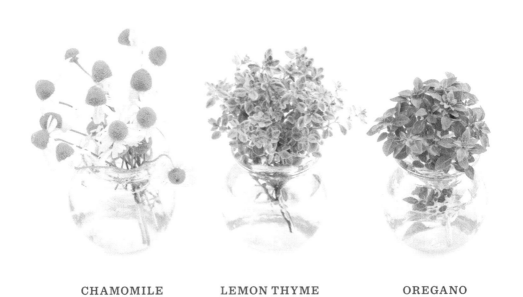

CHAMOMILE   LEMON THYME   OREGANO

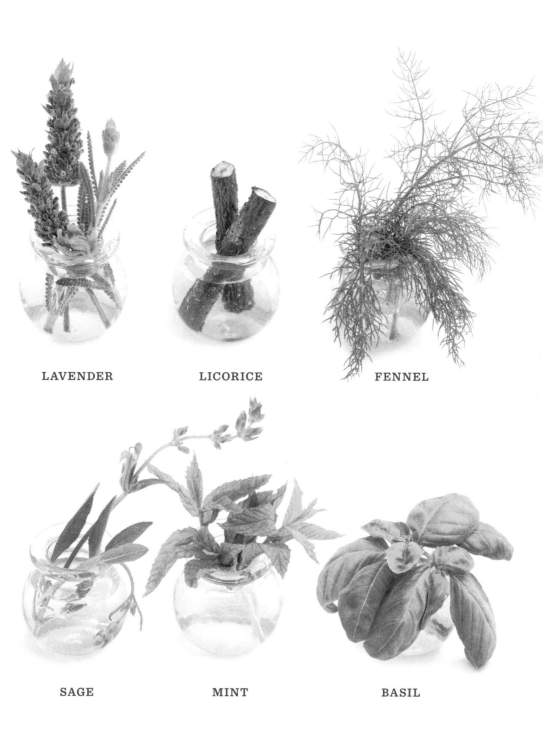

LAVENDER LICORICE FENNEL

SAGE MINT BASIL

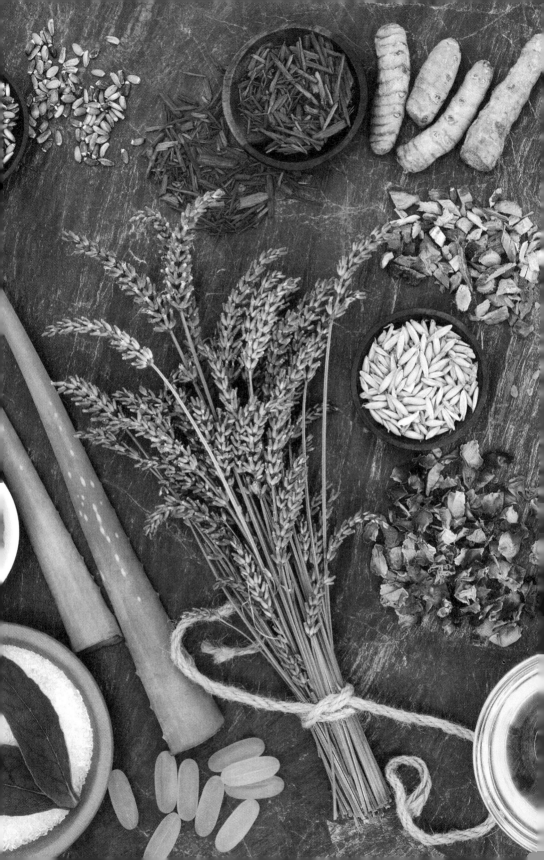

Chapter 1

Historical Use of Essential Oils

Essential oils are best known for their use in aromatherapy, where the inhaled oil's molecules stimulate the brain and impart physical and psychological properties. When applied topically, they are absorbed through the skin and into the bloodstream. They also pair well with many other treatments, such as massage, reflexology, reiki, herbal medicine, acupuncture, homeopathic remedies, and yoga. Concentrated organic elements with strong medicinal qualities, they are among the most powerful healing agents the natural environment has to offer. They have multiple uses: scenting soaps, candles, incense, and other products. Cinnamon, Peppermint, and Vanilla essential oils are used for flavoring food. They are also useful in the household, where you can concoct your own nontoxic cleansers and insect repellents to keep your spaces fresh and your body free of insect bites in a pure, natural way.

Pure essential oils are highly concentrated and deliciously aromatic compounds that have been pressed or distilled from plants. Essential oils are drawn from different parts of plants: the blossom, the fruit, the leaf, the stem, the bark, the wood, the roots, and the resin. They are called "essential" because they carry the essence of the plant, coming from deep within plant cells. Technically, they aren't oils at all; they don't contain fatty acids or any oily component. But they are complex compounds, as each essential oil comprises between 50 and 500 different naturally occurring chemicals.

We all love the wonderfully wide variety of natural aromas available from essential oils. Essential oils may have both positive and negative effects. For instance, one must be mindful about Cinnamon essential oil, which is an antiseptic and astringent, but also highly irritating to the skin.

Essential oils were highly valued in ancient times. In fact, the earliest evidence we have of their use as remedies is found as far back as 5000 BCE.

Anthropologists speculate that shamans first used aromatics by burning gums and resins for incense and doing smudging with aromatic plants, fragrant woods, barks, or herbs growing locally; these were the precursors of essential oils. The major aromatic trading centers would not appear for thousands of years. The best records of essential oils are found in the Middle East and in China.

In the 10th century, the Persians are generally credited with being the first to use distillation machines for extracting essential oils from plants in Mesopotamia, present-day Iraq. But there is some evidence that other ancient cultures—like the Egyptians, the Greeks, the Romans, the Chinese, and the Indians—also distilled essential oil–like extracts from plants long before that. It's possible that the oldest known uses of essential oils are in Ayurvedic medicine in India, but no one is sure exactly how old Ayurvedic medicine is.

The ancient Egyptians used essential oils for medicinal benefits, for spiritual enhancement, and as cosmetics. Cleopatra's legendary beauty was enhanced by many customary Egyptian beauty treatments, including essential oils, fatty oils, clays, and salts from the Dead Sea, the last famously brought to her by her lover Marc Antony.

Egyptians were famous for their mastery and use of aromatics and essential oils; these played an important role in their daily lives. They loved beauty and took great care of themselves. At festivals, the women wore on their heads perfumed cones, which would melt under the hot Egyptian sun and release a lovely aroma. They would also oil their bodies after bathing to prevent the drying of their skin and for its rejuvenating properties.

Around 48 BCE, when Julius Caesar and Cleopatra returned to Rome after conquering Egypt, bottles of aromatic fragrances were tossed into the crowd as a show of Roman dominion over Egypt.

Egyptian spirituality was the province of temple priests and priestesses, who basically worked as doctors. With their renowned herbal preparations, tinctures, unguents, salves, and ointments, they took care of the people's health. They also applied special fragrances and perfumes, both as part of their spiritual practices and for medicinal purposes. Many of their wide array of aromatic balms, resins, and powders are still valued and used today.

Ancient Egyptian temple murals depict the extraction of essential oils and also record recipes and formulas used by Egyptian royalty. When King Tutankhamen's tomb was opened in 1922, among all the wonderful things that were in there, there were over 50 ancient carved alabaster jars for essential oils. And the story goes that in previous raids of the tomb these essential oils were stolen but the gold was not touched! This shows how very valued essential oils were.

In 2650–2575 BCE Egypt, essential oils were also used in the mummification process. Studies reported by *National Geographic* have found the linen wrappings covering mummies to have been treated with resins from fir and pine trees, beeswax, myrrh, palm wine, cassia, camphor oil, and other substances that had drying or antibacterial properties. The studies used a combination of gas chromatography and mass spectrometry to examine tiny samples, and they found that most of the oils used were derived from plants.

Organic chemist Richard Evershed told *National Geographic* that "The embalmers really had to have a tremendous amount of knowledge about the properties of these materials and their ability to prevent rehydration and inhibit microbial growth to truly protect the bodies over a long period of time." He studied 13 mummies dating from roughly 1985 BCE to 395 CE. They used frankincense, myrrh, galbanum, cinnamon, cedarwood, juniper berry, and spikenard to preserve the bodies of their royalty in preparation for the afterlife. These valuable herbs and spices were laboriously transported across inhospitable deserts by Arab merchants to distribute to Assyria, Babylon, China, Egypt, Greece, Rome, and Persia. The most prized were frankincense and myrrh. Because demand outstripped supply during those early trading years, these herbs and spices had huge value.

The Egyptians' rich botanical knowledge was assimilated by the Assyrians, the Babylonians, the Hebrews, the Greeks, and the Romans, who all borrowed from Egypt's huge knowledge of aromatic medicine.

In Greece, after Alexander the Great's invasion of Egypt in the third century BCE, the use of aromatics, herbs, and perfumes became much more common. This prompted great interest in all things fragrant. Hippocrates (circa 460–377 BCE), considered the father of modern medicine, studied and documented the medicinal effects of over 300 plants. In his treatments, he would typically employ baths, massage with infusions, or the ingestion of herbs such as fennel, parsley, hypericum, or valerian. He was one of the first to regard the entire body as one organism. He understood that externally applied essential oils are absorbed into our system and affect our internal organs. This belief, known as "holism," is one of the fundamental principles of therapeutic aromatherapy. Hippocrates also believed that surgery should be used only as a last resort. He thought aromatics were so useful that he had Athens fumigated with them to combat the plague. He even treated fallen soldiers on the battlefields with aromatics.

A contemporary of Hippocrates, Theophrastus of Athens (circa 371–287 BCE) was also a philosopher and student of Aristotle. He investigated everything about plants and even how scents affected the emotions. Generally referred to today as the founder of botany, he wrote several volumes on the subject, including *The History of Plants*, which became one of the most important botanical science references for centuries to come.

> *"It is to be expected the perfumes should have medicinal properties in view of the virtues of their spices. The effect of plasters and of what some may call poultices prove these virtues, since they disperse tumors and abscesses and produce a distinct effect on the body and its interior parts."*
>
> —Theophrastus

A few centuries later, the Greek physician Dioscorides (circa 40–90 CE) wrote the *Material Medical*, a monumental reference book on herbs and pharmacy. He compiled the material while traveling throughout the Roman empire with Emperor Nero's army, collecting samples of the local medicinal herbs everywhere he went. *Material Medical* cites many of the herbs and essential oils we use today, like cardamom, cinnamon, myrrh, basil, fennel, frankincense, juniper, pine, rose, rosemary, and thyme. Bay laurel was used to produce a trancelike state; rose, myrtle, and coriander were respected for their aphrodisiac properties; myrrh and marjoram were used as sedatives. Myrrh was also helpful in relieving gum infections; juniper berry as a diuretic; and cypress in relieving diarrhea. Scented ointments and oils were recognized as having great physical and psychological benefits.

Essential oils figure prominently in Ayurvedic medicine, which has been practiced for approximately 5,000 years. These oils are mainly applied with massage. Records dating from 2000 BCE describe patients being prescribed Cinnamon, Ginger, Myrrh, Coriander, Spikenard, and Sandalwood oils by their doctors. Jasmine was prescribed as a general tonic for the entire body, and rose as an antidepressant and to fortify the liver. Chamomile was used as a remedy for headaches, dizziness, and colds. Basil was valued as a sacred plant that would open the heart and mind, bestowing love and devotion. In the Vedas, the most sacred book of India, over 700 herbs and aromatic plants are listed, together with their therapeutic and spiritual uses. For the most part, many of the properties ascribed to the herbs and aromatic oils by the ancients have been confirmed by science today.

Deeply influenced by the Greeks, Roman culture used aromatic materials and essential oils lavishly, probably more than any other culture. The Romans incorporated them in baths and massages several times a day, scenting their bodies, their hair, and even their beds. The most exotic of these oils were used to make highly valued fragrances.

In China, herb and plant medicine is an integral part of traditional medicine. Specific use of essential oils can be traced back to *Shennong Bencaojing*, the oldest surviving medical text, dated around 2700 BCE. It was recorded by the emperor Shennong, considered to be the father of Chinese herbal medicine and traditional Chinese medicine; he is also said to have discovered tea and acupuncture. Shennong recorded the information he gathered on 365 herbal plants, including their properties and uses. He apparently tested these plants on himself. This suggests that the Chinese may even have preceded the Egyptians in their use and knowledge of plant-based medicines.

Huángdì, the Yellow Emperor, is another important influence. He is said to have written the Yellow Emperor's *Classic of Internal Medicine* in 2697 BCE. This book on internal medicine covers essential oils, which are still used by practitioners today.

The knowledge of distillation and isolation of essential oils spread thoughout Europe and was recorded in the period from the 11th to the 13th centuries. These distilled oils became a specialty of the medieval European pharmacies. By about 1500 CE, Europeans were being treated with oils of Cedarwood, Calamus, Costus, Rose, Rosemary, Spike, Incense, Turpentine, Sage, Cinnamon, Benzoin, and Myrrh.

The Swiss physician Paracelsus played an important role in stimulating physicians and pharmacists to seek essential oils from aromatic leaves, woods, and roots.

> *"The art of healing comes from nature, not from the physician. Therefore the physician must start from nature, with an open mind."*
>
> —Paracelsus

But during the Middle Ages the Catholic Church denounced the use of aromatics as decadent, proclaiming the practice of using herbs and essential oils to be witchcraft. Fortunately, monks of the era retained their knowledge of these substances' medicinal uses. The church's ban temporarily reduced the use of essential oils therapeutically, but they were still used for their fragrance.

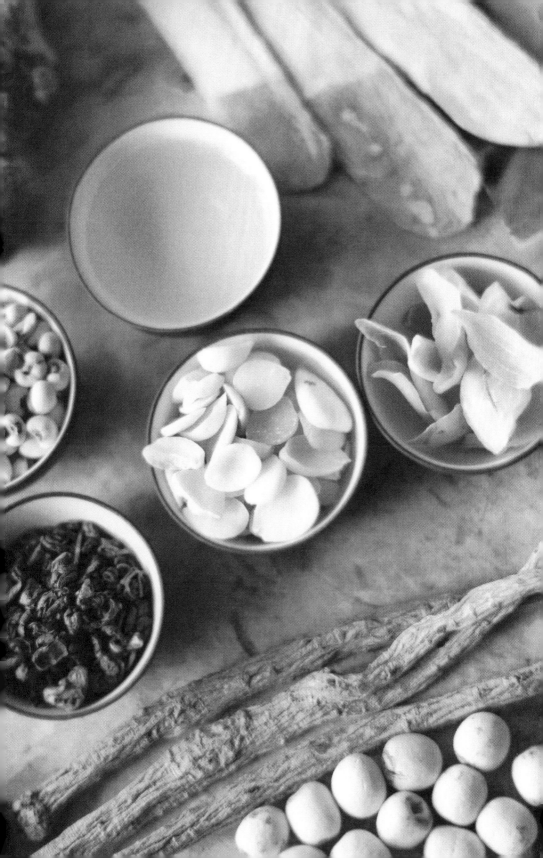

By the 1600s, a new era of progress was dawning, with the spread of knowledge through printed books about essential oils and herbal medicine that were now readily available. Many books about the distillation of essential oils were written in the 16th century, especially in Germany, which appeared to be the center of a European aromatherapy renaissance. Hieronymus Brunschwig, a German physician, wrote several very successful books on essential oil distillation that were translated into every European language. In 1597 he referenced 25 essential oils, including Rosemary, Lavender, Clove, Cinnamon, Myrrh, and Nutmeg. By the middle of the 18th century in Europe, about 100 essential oils had been introduced.

During the 1800s, patients in England, Germany, and France were being prescribed essential oils. At this time in southern France there were large flower-growing districts, and during tuberculosis bouts, workers processing flowers and herbs generally remained disease-free. This led to the first recorded lab test of the antibacterial properties of essential oils in 1887.

In 1910 French cosmetic chemist René-Maurice Gattefossé was badly burned in a lab accident. He quickly submerged both his arms in a container of Lavender oil and saw immediate results. This astonishing healing experience led Gattefossé to explore the medical uses of essential oils by treating soldiers during World War I. After the war, he continued the same work and coined the term *aromatherapie*—the treatment of disease and injury with essential oils—and published his book by the same name in 1937.

In the early 1930s, Austrian-born biochemist and nurse Marguerite Maury lectured and gave seminars throughout Europe, promoting the health-giving and rejuvenating properties of essential oils.

During France's Indochina War (1946–54), Jean Valnet, a colleague of Gattefossé's, began to use essential oils as antiseptics for wounded soldiers. The story goes that Valnet was treating the wounded and ran out of antibiotics. In desperation he used essential oils and was amazed to see how well the essential oils fought infection. He continued to use them afterwards, and in 1964 he published his book, *The Practice of Aromatherapy*, a world-renowned reference on the subject.

Today, with the continuing spread of knowledge about essential oils, many people are discovering, or rediscovering, this powerful medicine. All around the world people are using essential oils to enhance their health and well-being, whether through aromatherapy, experiences of beauty through smell and taste, or to treat ailments. Hopefully, we will preserve the insights from ancient cultures and continue to discover new ones.

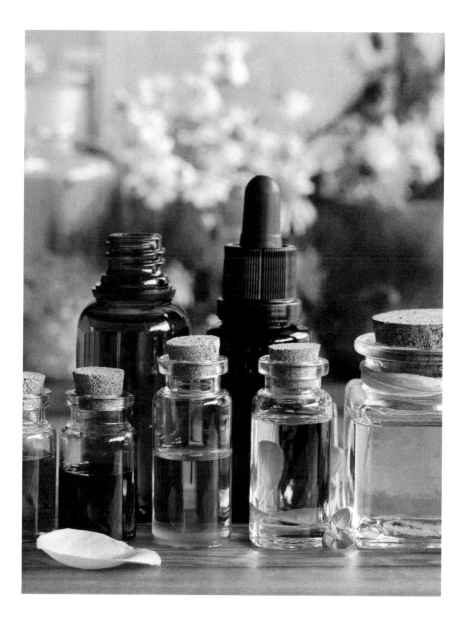

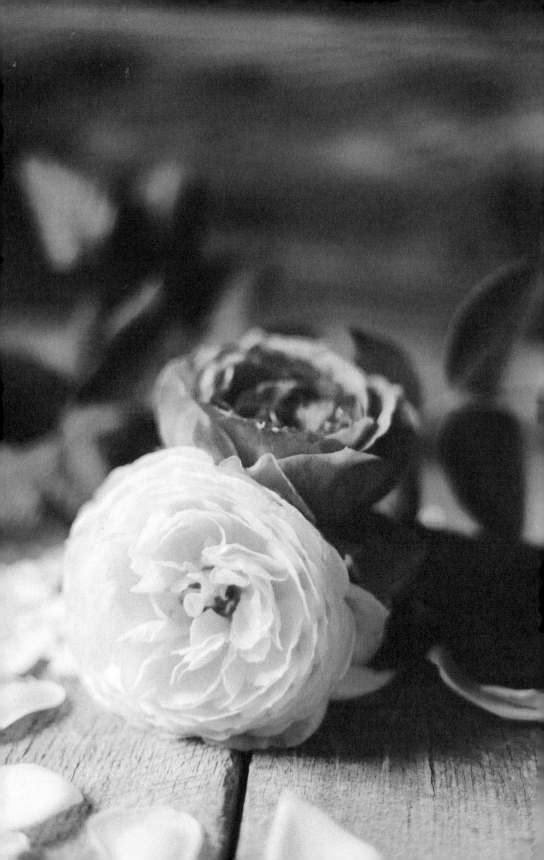

Chapter 2

Benefits of Essential Oils

HOW THEY WORK

Essential oils are a natural way to prevent and treat ailments. They play an important role in complementary medicine healing; help stop the growth of bacteria, viruses, and fungi; and promote general well-being. They remedy conditions ranging from depression to infections. And they can be used in a variety of ways to treat a wide range of ailments. They often work very well to alleviate chronic conditions like arthritis, tendinitis, and rheumatism. Single essential oils have many uses; they work for multiple ailments, not just one or two. Plus, there are hundreds of essential oils to choose from. Keep in mind that if you are allergic to a particular plant, you will most likely be allergic to the essential oil made from that plant.

HOW THEY ARE MADE

Essential oil extraction is much like winemaking—it's both an art and a science. There are at least five different techniques for this. The method used generally depends on the distiller's experience and the oil's intended use.

Essential oils are highly concentrated. It takes 100 pounds of lavender flowers and 2 tons of Bulgarian roses to produce just a single pound of both Lavender essential oil and Rose essential oil, respectively. Imagine: One single drop of essential oil is the gathered essence of hundreds of flowers or plants!

One drop of essential oil has the same concentration of plant essence as around 30 cups of herbal tea!

The essential oil molecules come from deep within the plant, inside small sacs. When you rub lavender, rosemary, or sage leaves or flowers with your fingers, these sacs burst and release minuscule essential oil molecules, and that's how you get their delicious, natural aroma.

Steam Distillation

The most common method of extraction used to make the most frequently used essential oils—including Lavender, Peppermint, and Eucalyptus—is steam dilation. Most essential oils are distilled in a brief process, except Ylang-ylang, which takes 22 hours to complete.

There are two types of steam distillation.

1 STEAM: The plant parts are placed into a tightly sealed chamber into which steam is injected. The steam hits the plants, and this heat makes the small sacs holding the essential oil burst. Essential oil molecules are tiny and easily move with the steam out into a chilled condenser. Once the collection is complete, the essential oil and the water are separated using a centrifuge, leaving behind the pure essential oil.

2 WATER AND STEAM: The whole plant is placed above boiling water, the steam rises through it, gathering the essential oil molecules. The steam continues up with the essential oil molecules into another receptacle that pushes the oil and steam through a final separator of water and essential oil.

In both methods, the extracted scented water, called hydrosol, is saved and used to add fragrance to linen sprays, perfumes, body lotion, facial moisturizers, and the like.

This gentle heat method of distillation works best on essential oils that release components only after a certain amount of exposure to heat. For example, German chamomile has been found to release its anti-inflammatory component, chamulzine, only through distillation. This is what gives this essential oil its characteristic blue color.

Carbon Dioxide Extraction

There are four methods of carbon dioxide extraction. The two most common are carbon dioxide distillation and supercritical carbon dioxide distillation.

1   CARBON DIOXIDE DISTILLATION, OR CO_2 EXTRACTION, is very similar to cold-pressing in that it doesn't use any heat to extract the essential oil. As a result, the extracted oils are not even slightly altered. The carbon dioxide carries the essential oil away from the raw plant material. The carbon dioxide is chilled and then blasted through the plant material.

2   SUPERCRITICAL CO_2 DISTILLATION is used mostly with Frankincense, Myrrh, and Calendula essential oils, and spicy-smelling oils from cloves, black peppers, and gingers. The carbon dioxide is heated and then blown through the plant matter at a much higher speed than the previous extraction method. This transforms the carbon dioxide into a heavy vapor, which quickly carries the essential oil away. As the carbon dioxide is not hot, the essential oil remains unaltered.

There are two more carbon dioxide distillation methods that yield even more highly concentrated essential oils: CO_2 Totals and CO_2 Selects. They are both labeled as CO_2 Extracted, with the distinction apparent in their consistencies. One should dilute them by 50–60 percent before use.

1   CO_2 TOTALS are called "totals" because they use large amounts of the plant matter, including the resins, waxes, and color compounds that normally are discarded. Therefore, CO_2 Totals generally need to be heated to be poured, as they are pasty or waxy.

2   THE CO_2 SELECTS method produces essential oils that are also thicker than most other essential oils because they also keep parts of the plant's natural waxes, resins, and color compounds in the finished product. Unlike CO₂ Totals, however, these don't need to be heated before use.

Citrus Fruits Cold-Pressing

This method is used exclusively with citrus fruits. Cold-pressing, or expression, is a simple method—you place the aromatic part of the fruit rind in a press at 120°F and *voilà*!

Hot Effleurage

This is the original and oldest-known process of oil extraction. In hot effleurage, you place petals in a shallow layer of warm fatty oil and this absorbs the essential oils from the petals. As the flowers wilt, you keep placing new layers on top, until the oil is completely saturated with essential oil. You then extract the essential oil by soaking the material in 50 percent alcohol. You can then use the leftover fat or oil to scent soaps and similar products. This method is rarely used today, except by exclusive perfume manufacturers.

Solvent Extraction

This method uses chemical solvents, such as methylene chloride, hexane, or benzene, instead of water or carbon dioxide, to extract essential oils. Most of the chemicals evaporate during the first phase of the extraction. Then the rest are spun off in a centrifuge or vacuumed away. What remains after this process are minute traces in the essential oil. There is disagreement about whether these traces, albeit minute, are acceptable for use in aromatherapy. The renowned aromatherapist Robert Tisserand is one of many practitioners who are not convinced that this method produces the healthiest essential oil.

Solvent extraction produces essential oils called "absolutes," such as Rose, Jasmine, Tuberose, Carnation, Gardenia, Jonquil, Violet Leaf, Narcissus, Mimosa, and other delicate flowers. Both Neroli and Rose oils can either be distilled or solvent-extracted. Absolutes are used by therapists for their psychological properties to elevate mood, and they are also commonly used on animals, especially horses.

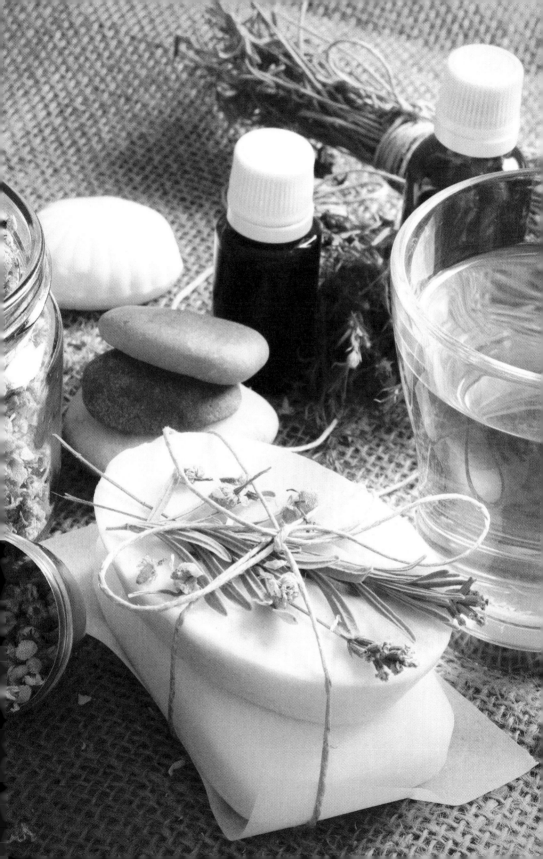

Some Benefits of Essential Oils When Used Topically and for Aromatherapy

Name	Part of the Plant	How to Use	Spiritual & Health Benefits	Caution with/ Avoid if
Basil*	leaf	Topical— Inhaled	Clarifying—Antimicrobial	Pregnant
Bergamot	peel	Topical— Inhaled	Uplifting—Antidepressant	Direct sun
Cajeput	leaf	Topical— Inhaled	Clarity—Psoriasis, bronchitis	Sensitive skin
Cardamom	seed	Topical— Inhaled	Aphrodisiac—Stomachaches	None
Carrot Seed	seed	Topical— Inhaled	Opens third eye—Blood cleanser	Pregnant
Cedarwood	wood	Topical— Inhaled	Calming—Astringent	Pregnant
Celery	seed	Topical— Inhaled	Alleviates grief & anxiety— Diuretic	Pregnant
Chamomile	flower	Topical— Inhaled	For impatience—Anti-allergic	Pregnant
Cinnamon	bark	Topical— Inhaled	Aphrodisiac—Digestive issues	Pregnant
Citronella	grass	Topical— Inhaled	Inner vision—Headaches	Sensitive skin
Clary Sage	flower	Topical— Inhaled	Euphoric—Menstrual cramps	Pregnant
Clovebud	flower	Topical— Inhaled	Energizing—Toothache	Pregnant
Cypress	needle	Topical— Inhaled	Comfort—Varicose veins	Pregnant
Elemi	resin	Topical— Inhaled	Soul protecting—Urinary tract	None
Eucalyptus	leaf	Topical— Inhaled	Calming—Respiratory tract	None

*These essential oils are toxic in high concentrations.

Name	Part of the Plant	How to Use	Spiritual & Health Benefits	Caution with/ Avoid if
Eucalyptus Lemon	leaf	Topical— Inhaled	Alleviates hypersensitivity— Diabetes	None
Fennel*	seed	Topical— Inhaled	Purifying—Hormone balancer	Prone to seizures— Pregnant
Fir Needle	needle	Topical— Inhaled	Inspiration—Muscle aches	None
Frankincense	resin	Topical— Inhaled	Spirituality—Aging skin	None
Galbanum	resin	Topical— Inhaled	Grounding—Lung infections	Pregnant
Geranium	flower	Topical— Inhaled	Promotes peace—Addictions	Pregnant
Ginger	rhizome	Topical— Inhaled	Opens to love—Antispasmodic	Sensitive skin
Grapefruit	peel	Topical— Inhaled	Happiness—Cellulite, diuretic	Direct sun
Helichrysum	flower	Topical— Inhaled	Meditation—Regenerating cells	None
Hyssop*	flower	Topical— Inhaled	Negativity—Regulates blood pressure	Prone to seizures— Pregnant
Jasmine	flower	Topical— Inhaled	Forgiveness—Prostate	Pregnant
Lavandin	flower	Topical— Inhaled	Patience with self—Arthritis	None
Lavender	flower	Topical— Inhaled	Inspiration—Palpitations	Pregnant
Lemon	peel	Topical— Inhaled	Vitality—Detoxifies liver, kidneys	Direct sun

Name	Part of the Plant	How to Use	Spiritual & Health Benefits	Caution with/ Avoid If
Lemongrass	leaf	Topical— Inhaled	Removes obstacles—Acne	Sensitive skin
Lime	peel	Topical— Inhaled	Releases trauma—Antibiotic	Direct sun
Litsea	fruit	Topical— Inhaled	Connects to inner child—Heart	Sensitive skin
Mandarin	peel	Topical— Inhaled	Boosts inner child—Promotes sleep	Direct sun
Melissa	flower	Topical— Inhaled	Opens the heart—Heart	Sensitive skin
Myrrh	resin	Topical— Inhaled	Releases trauma—Wrinkles	Pregnant
Myrtle	leaf	Topical— Inhaled	Unconditional love—Asthma	None
Neroli	flower	Topical— Inhaled	Opens the heart—Insomnia	None
Niaouli	leaf	Topical— Inhaled	Healing—Regulates white blood count	None
Nutmeg*	seed	Topical— Inhaled	Prosperity—Eliminates toxins	Pregnant
Orange	peel	Topical— Inhaled	Centering—Lowers cholesterol	Direct sun
Orange, Blood	peel	Topical— Inhaled	Luck—Fibromyalgia	Direct sun
Oregano*	leaf	Topical— Inhaled	Purifying—Prevents diseases	Children— Pregnant
Palmarosa	grass	Topical— Inhaled	Opens to love—Mature skin	High blood pressure
Patchouli	leaf	Topical— Inhaled	For attraction—Loss of appetite	None
Peppermint	leaf	Topical— Inhaled	Dispels pride—Lowers fevers	Pregnant
Petitgrain	leaf	Topical— Inhaled	Tempers obsessiveness—Candida	None

Name	Part of the Plant	How to Use	Spiritual & Health Benefits	Caution with/ Avoid if
Pine	leaf	Topical— Inhaled	Boosts will to live—Gallstones	None
Ravintsara	leaf	Topical— Inhaled	Fearlessness—Chronic fatigue	Pregnant
Rose Absolute	flower	Topical— Inhaled	Creativity—Alleviates menopausal symptoms	Pregnant
Rose Otto	flower	Topical— Inhaled	Blessing—Hangovers	Pregnant
Sage*	leaf	Topical— Inhaled	Focus—Raises blood pressure	Prone to seizures— Pregnant
Sandalwood	wood	Topical— Inhaled	Meditation—Cystitis, kidneys	None
Spearmint	leaf	Topical— Inhaled	Heals the soul—Migraines	Pregnant
Spikenard	root	Topical— Inhaled	Releases the past—Detoxifying	None
Spruce	needle	Topical— Inhaled	Communication—Skin toner	None
Tangerine	peel	Topical— Inhaled	Spiritual—Aids circulation	Direct sun
Tea Tree	leaf	Topical— Inhaled	Energizing—Children's diseases	None
Tulsi*	leaf	Topical— Inhaled	Dispels fear—Heart disease	Pregnant
Valerian	root	Topical— Inhaled	Dispels panic—Sedative	Pregnant
Vanilla	bean	Topical— Inhaled	Spirituality—Aphrodisiac	None
Vetiver	root	Topical— Inhaled	Protection—Immune system	None
Ylang-ylang	flower	Topical— Inhaled	Acceptance—Infertility	None

Application Methods of Essential Oils

Here are some general guidelines for using essential oils. Be aware that application methods vary for each essential oil, so be sure to check the specifications before proceeding.

TOPICAL USE

10 drops essential oil in 1 ounce carrier oil, massage oil, or lotion

Apply to skin or in bathwater.

Carrier oils, which are dilution agents for essential oils, are usually a natural vegetable, nut, or seed oil, excellent for massage and to nourish and moisturize the skin while imparting the essential oil's specific benefits.

CARRIER OIL: A dilution agent that should be used with essential oils before application or use. Examples include olive oil, avocado oil, almond oil, and castor oil.

INHALATION METHOD

4 drops essential oil in 2 cups hot water

Pour water into a bowl for steam. Cover your head with a towel, and breathe in. Start gently. You can also use an essential oil diffuser.

✳

It's easy to get started with essential oils as they are so handy, versatile, portable, potent, and safe! Now that you understand the basics of essential oils, let's move on to how to use them . . .

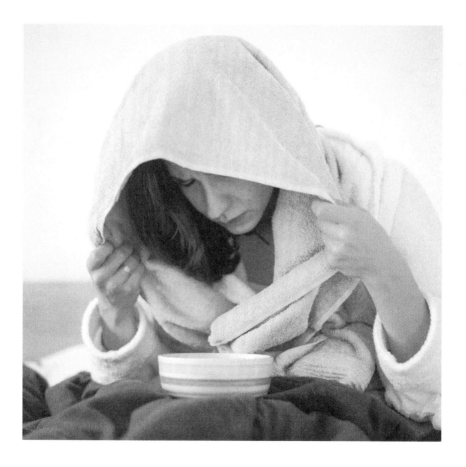

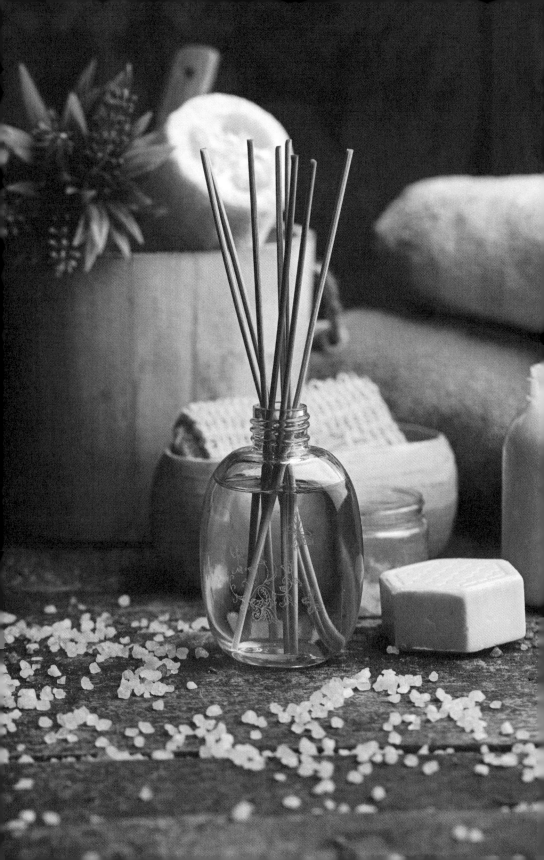

Chapter 3

How to Use Essential Oils

Essential oils have many uses, including as first-aid remedies, for treating minor illnesses, adding to body care products (lotion, shampoo, conditioner), as insect repellents, and as natural air fresheners.

Whenever possible, use only pure organic essential oils; avoid synthetic fragrances. When shopping for them, watch out for phrases such as *fragrance oil, nature identical oil,* and *perfume oil.* None of these indicate a pure, single essential oil, and some even have chemicals. Organic essential oils are grown without herbicides and pesticides. Because plants *do* absorb these substances, it follows that we will breathe/absorb these chemicals into our system when we use them.

Some companies market their essential oils with terms such as *therapeutic grade, food grade, aromatherapy grade, medicinal grade,* or label them certified. But there is no formally approved grading standard system in the essential oil industry. These terms vary from company to company, and some are used merely as a marketing ploy. Not all companies use these terms with intentional deception in mind. If you're looking at a product from a reputable company, then you can likely trust the company's grading system to be genuine. Also, check if the company's products are gas chromatography– and mass spectrometry–tested, and make sure they are not in plastic bottles, but in dark-colored glass bottles. Stay away from much cheaper oils; most honest companies price the same type of essential oil within a few dollars.

In labeling an essential oil as a *therapeutic grade oil,* companies mean that:

* It's distilled without using chemicals.

* It's more expensive to produce because it requires hundreds of pounds of plant material to distill only a single pound of oil.

* It's sourced from plants grown in a native indigenous environment.

Food-grade essential oil means that it's listed by the Food and Drug Administration as one of the "substances generally recognized as safe." But that doesn't mean it's edible: the FDA also places chemicals, synthetic flavorings, and natural extracts on the same list.

Essential oils are generally administered either aromatically or topically. The most common way to apply essential oils is topically, meaning it's generally absorbed through the skin and breathed in during a message. Aromatic applications are inhaled as either single or blended oils. Pick the method you prefer and the oil you need. Keep in mind that in some methods you inhale or absorb more essential oils than in others.

INDIRECT INHALATION

Diffusion is the simplest, most common method of applying aromatics. Essential oil diffusers are versatile and easy to use.

Best are cold-air diffusers. They use ultrasonic vibrations that break the tiny oil particles into a mist that remains suspended in the air for hours. Their aroma fills the atmosphere and breathing them in has specific physical and/or emotional benefits.

CAUTION: Follow manufacturer's instructions or you could clog your diffuser by using water, vegetable oil, or undiluted essential oils.

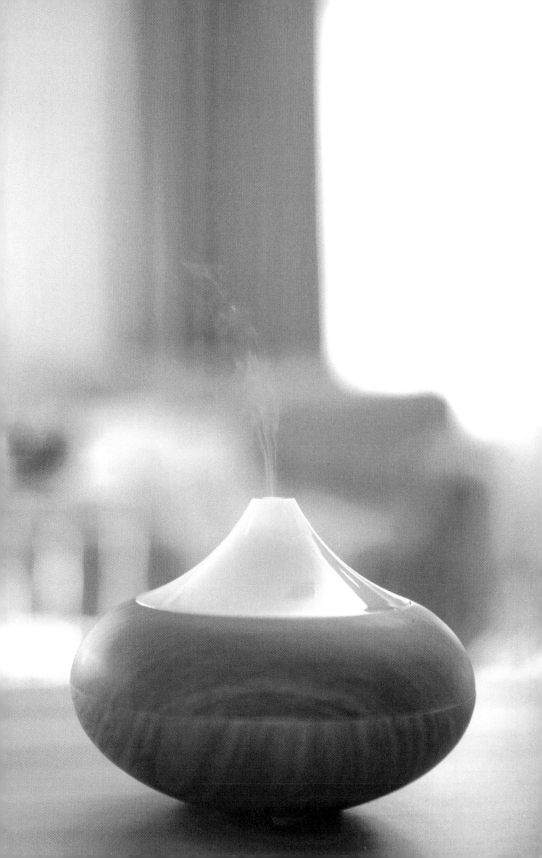

Humidifiers, vaporizers, vents, or fans are all good alternatives if you don't have a diffuser around, especially in hotels, offices, and cars. They're great for allergies and sinuses in the winter.

Put a few drops of oil on a cloth or cotton ball and place the cloth or cotton ball in front of the diffuser's valve.

CAUTION: Don't put the oil directly on the apparatus. Oil causes the plastic parts to get sticky or to degrade over time.

Hot water vapors are excellent for colds, respiratory issues, sore throats, irritation, dryness, allergies, and congestion.

Put 3–5 drops of oil in a bowl of very hot water. With your head and shoulders covered with a large towel and your eyes closed, bend over the bowl and breathe in the steam for as long as it lasts (a minimum of 1 minute). Pull up to breathe fresh air whenever you need to.

CAUTION: Don't use water that's too hot; steam can burn your nasal passages. If you're feeling dizzy or nauseous, stop immediately.

DIRECT INHALATION

A simple, direct, and effective method with immediate benefit.

Sit or lie in a comfortable position. Put a few drops of oil in the palm of your hand, rub your hands together, cup them over your nose and mouth, and breathe in very deeply 3–5 times. Relax for 3 minutes afterwards.

CAUTION: Don't directly inhale Cinnamon or Clove oils. Unless specifically blended to diffuse, they are strong and spicy and can burn your airways. Only pick oils that are suitable for direct inhalation. See table on page 16.

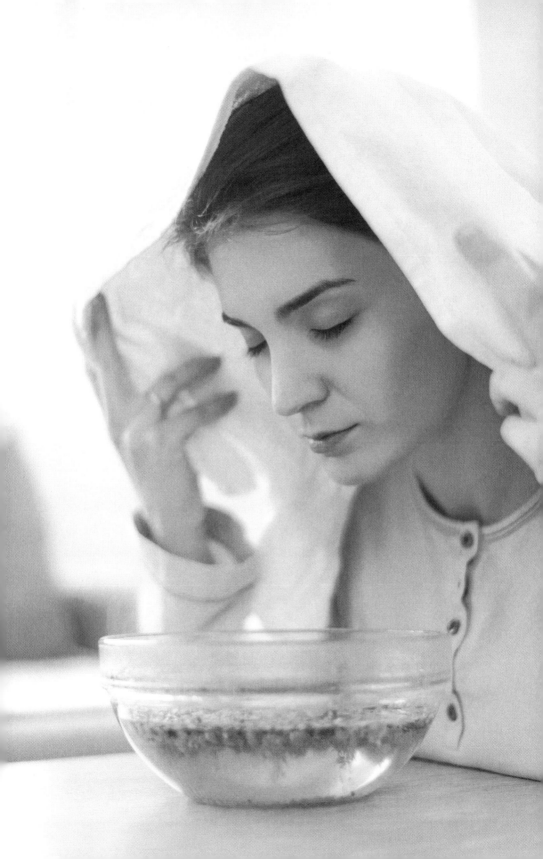

INTERNAL USE

Essential oils must be treated with caution, as they are highly concentrated.

For internal use, only use therapeutic grade oils from a trustworthy company. They shouldn't be taken internally except by those well versed in their uses, since not all oils are safe to ingest.

Essential oils are also used in cooking. In French aromatherapy they use carefully prepared compounds for ingestion.

The quantity for internal use is from 1 to 3 drops per dose, taking into account the illness, the patient's profile, and the patient's requirements. Generally diluted with warm water, soy or rice milk, or placed in a capsule. Use only on temporary basis, not for prolonged use.

Frequently used for treating infectious diseases, requiring a high dose, and only under the supervision of a certified aromatherapist.

CAUTION: Oregano and Cinnamon oils can cause stinging or burning, and damage the mouth and esophagus. They can be poisonous or toxic in high concentrations. If not administered correctly, they can cause a stinging sensation in the mouth, indigestion, and chest pains. Taking multiple essential oils internally on a daily basis can be damaging to the liver, kidneys, stomach, and intestines.

Topical applications are oils absorbed directly through the skin into the bloodstream. For example, you can apply oil on specific points in reflexology.

ACUPRESSURE

Acupressure is acupuncture without the needles. Apply the oil to the acupressure point; the combination of both the pressure point and the oil is effective.

CAUTION: Even though acupressure is simple, before you practice it, read up on it to make sure you don't damage the body's delicate underlying structures.

You could also recommend the use of essential oils to your local certified acupuncturist.

Bath and Shower

In baths or showers, the oils easily penetrate the skin and are absorbed. You also benefit from indirect inhalation.

Make your own body washes, shampoos, and conditioners by adding 12–15 drops of oil per ounce of product.

Add 3–6 drops of oil to running bathwater and soak. Mix with a carrier oil and you won't need to moisturize afterwards.

In the shower, place 3–5 drops of oil on a damp washcloth, place on your chest or on the floor. Afterwards, rub your body with it, making gentle circular movements working your way toward your heart.

COLD PACKS AND HOT COMPRESSES

Cold packs and hot compresses reduce inflammation from strains and sprains, soothe headaches, ease sinuses, help with fever, and relax muscle cramps.

Keep cold packs in place no longer than 20 minutes. Usually made of fabric filled with rice or buckwheat and dabbed with 8–10 drops of oil. Refreeze after use and periodically refresh with a few new drops.

Hot compresses are ideal for treating pain, including chronic muscle discomfort, rheumatism, menstrual cramps, and toothaches. They are made with a small towel, water, and 4–5 drops of oil. Leave on until they reach body temperature. Either place the compress on the affected area or rub the oil onto the skin and then cover with the compress.

CAUTION: Don't use on tender or broken skin, and use carefully on areas with poor circulation.

LAYERING ESSENTIAL OILS

Layering essential oils is different from creating a blend. By layering oils, you can treat more than one issue at a time.

Apply oil to the area, using 1 or 2 drops. Once absorbed, apply a second layer of a different oil on top, and continue layering oils, depending on why you're using them.

For a sprain, for instance, apply a layer for the pain, a layer for the swelling, and a third layer for the bruising. See chapter 4 for details on the most popular essential oils and their uses.

CAUTION: If you ever get essential oil in your eyes or onto your mucous membranes, rinse the affected area with milk to neutralize the oil.

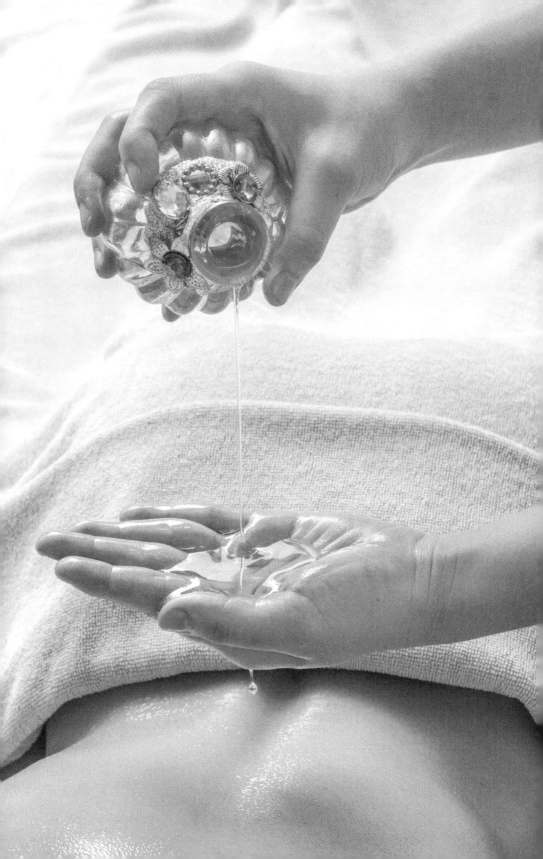

MASSAGING WITH ESSENTIAL OILS

Massaging with essential oils maximizes the healing potential.

Add 12–15 drops of oil per ounce of good carrier oil. Bring your massage oil with you to your therapist.

CAUTION: Even though essential oils are well diluted during a massage, always check the safety indication of each before using. For instance, citrus oils mustn't be used before exposure to UV light because they increase photosensitivity so you may be more likely to sunburn or experience skin discoloration.

DIRECT APPLICATION OF ESSENTIAL OILS

Direct application is for pain relief or antibacterial protection for cuts, bruises, fungal infections, rashes, burns, and insect bites.

Apply blended in carrier oil, or, as pure oils, sprays, salves, and ointments.

As you see, essential oils are easy to use, so enjoy their multiple uses!

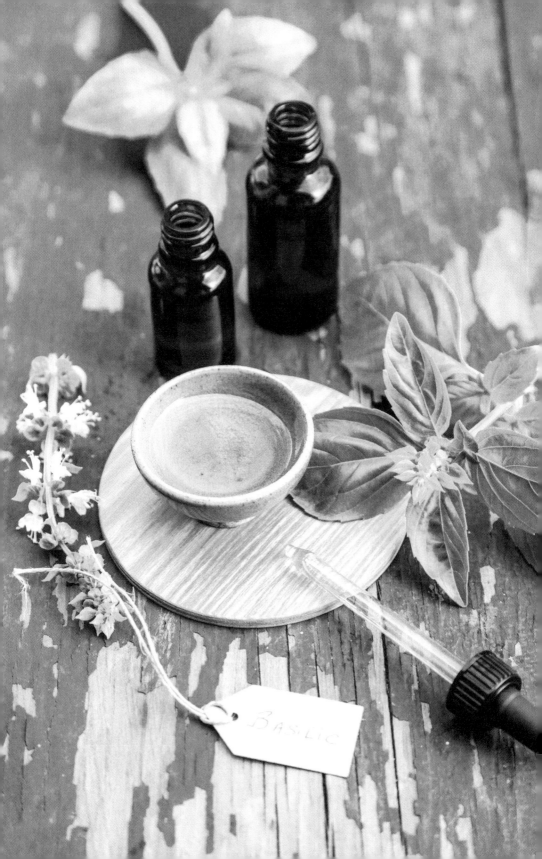

Chapter 4

The Most Popular Essential Oils

There are many wonderful essential oils out there to choose from. In this chapter, I have narrowed down my top picks and highlighted the best qualities of each oil so that you can find one best suited to your needs.

Keep in mind that care should be taken when applying essential oils to the skin. They are highly concentrated and most should be diluted before topical application. Unless otherwise stated, it is best to dilute the oils with a carrier oil to a concentration of no more than 3 percent of the overall volume of each oil. Reduce this by at least half if you are making a blend for children.

If you are looking for oils that boost circulation, and, subsequently, detoxification, look for oils that are classified as "warming" in nature. These oils not only speed the flow of blood to the area applied, they also bolster the health of the internal organs.

ANGELICA

Angelica archangelica

Angelica is good for clearing skin that is dull or irritated. It is useful in detoxifying the body and treating arthritis, gout, coughs, bronchitis, indigestion, and many stress-related disorders. It acts as a slight diuretic and helps to improve energy levels.

ANISE, STAR

Illicium verum

This is best used for sore and stiff muscles, and for help in reducing rheumatic pain. It is effective at treating coughs and bronchitis and is a boon for addressing digestive system disorders, such as indigestion and flatulence.

ASAFETIDA

Ferula asafoetida

This is especially useful when diffused to ease coughs, bronchitis, and asthma. It also helps pep you up and reduces stress.

BASIL

Ocimum basilicum

Basil makes a great insect repellent and can be used to ease the itch of insect bites. It helps ease sore and stiff muscles, gout, and rheumatism. Its strong antiviral and antimicrobial properties make it effective in treating respiratory-tract infections. It helps heal earaches as well. Rub into the abdomen to alleviate nausea, flatulence, and dyspepsia.

It should not be used by women who are pregnant, as it can cause a miscarriage.

BENZOIN

Styrax benzoin

Benzoin is great at reducing stress and tension. It helps to create a euphoric feeling, especially when combined with 3 drops of Jasmine or Rose oil.

It boosts circulation, soothes inflammation, and treats respiratory-tract infections. If you suffer from gout, Benzoin should be on your shopping list.

A MUST-HAVE OIL

BERGAMOT

Citrus bergamia

Bergamot is best known for its ability to ease depression and to lift the mood. It is also effective for thrush, pruritic, and many different skin conditions. It helps balance an oily complexion.

BLACK PEPPER

Piper nigrum

Black pepper is useful for treating neuralgia, stiff and sore muscles, and rheumatic pain. It helps to tone the muscles and boost the circulation. It is effective in the treatment of colds, flu, and viruses.

CARROT SEED

Daucus carota

Carrot Seed oil is extremely useful when it comes to treating skin conditions, such as eczema, dermatitis, rashes, and psoriasis. It is valuable for people with mature skin and to combat wrinkles. It helps to detoxify the body and can be useful when it comes to treating edema, gout, liver congestion, and a host of other conditions. Carrot Seed oil helps to regulate the menstrual cycle in women and eases the symptoms of PMS.

CEDARWOOD, ATLAS

Cedrus atlantica

Cedarwood is good for those with acne-prone and oily skin. It is also helpful in treating dermatitis, fungal infections, breakouts, eczema, and dandruff.

It can be rubbed into sore joints to alleviate arthritic pain.

It has strong antimicrobial and antiviral properties, making it a good remedy to fight colds, flu, nasal congestion, and bronchitis.

It is also a calming oil.

CELERY SEED

Apium graveolens

Celery seed is most useful for its ability to stimulate the lymphatic system. It is useful in treating rheumatism and gout. It assists in the treatment of indigestion and liver congestion.

For nursing mothers, it is useful in increasing the flow of milk. It has some analgesic properties as well.

A MUST-HAVE OIL

CHAMOMILE, ROMAN

Matricaria recutita

Chamomile is one of those oils that we should all have in our cabinet. It is extremely useful for calming a stressed mind and very effective at reducing inflammation and easing allergic reactions. It is the oil that is said to have the best analgesic properties of all.

CINNAMON

Cinnamomum zeylanicum

Although Cinnamon oil is useful, it can irritate the skin so it should be diluted extensively when applied topically. It is a warming oil that improves circulation and rheumatic pain.

It helps to rev up circulation and the digestive process and can help fight infections within the intestine. It is helpful when it comes to treating colds and flu.

Cinnamon oil should never be used by a pregnant woman, as it can stimulate uterine contractions.

CITRONELLA

Cymbopogon nardus

Citronella is best known for its properties as an insect repellent. If you want to boost its effectiveness in this area, mix with equal parts of Cedarwood oil and diffuse.

It is also useful in the treatment of colds, flu, headaches, and fatigue. If you battle with excessive perspiration, you can try mixing a drop or two of Citronella oil with cornstarch and applying it under your arms.

CLARY SAGE

Salvia officinalis

Clary Sage is best known for its effect on the nervous system. Extremely useful in reducing depression, stress, headaches, and nervous tension, it is also a valuable antispasmodic and can help relieve stiff and sore muscles. It can prevent hair loss and stave off wrinkles. It is best suited to those with oily skin.

CLOVE

Syzygium aromaticum

Clove is another oil that should be used in a weak dilution as it can irritate the skin. It is best known as a treatment for toothache but it has many other uses as well. It will help to treat respiratory-tract infections as well as asthma.

It eases sprained muscles and the pain of rheumatism and arthritis.

CORIANDER

Coriandrum sativum

Coriander is more than just a nice herb for cooking. It has a strong detoxifying action and can help to improve circulation. It helps to settle an upset stomach and fights all sorts of infections.

It will help you to overcome debility, neuralgia, migraines, and nervous exhaustion.

Coriander is also cilantro! After the coriander flowers and seeds, it is called coriander. *Cilantro* is Spanish for coriander leaves.

COSTUS

Saussurea costus

Costus has good antispasmodic properties and helps with stress-related illnesses.

CUMIN

Cuminum cyminum

Cumin is most useful as a detoxifying agent and as a means of improving circulation. It will help heal upsets in the digestive tract and soothe headaches and nervous exhaustion.

CYPRESS

Cupressus sempervirens

Cypress is useful for treating oily skin and excessive perspiration. It helps reduce the appearance of varicose veins and helps wounds to heal. It has strong antispasmodic properties and is a good pain reliever. It helps cure respiratory-tract infections and reduces anxiety related to stress.

DILL

Anethum graveolens

Dill is similar to fennel. It is excellent for treating bloating and edema. It helps to regulate a woman's periods and increases the flow of milk in nursing mothers.

ELEMI

Canarium luzonicum

Elemi is good for skin that is showing signs of aging and also at reducing inflammation. It will help heal infected cuts and respiratory-tract infections. It is a calming oil.

EUCALYPTUS

Eucalyptus globules

Eucalyptus oil helps heal skin infections (including those caused by lice), wounds, herpes, cuts, blisters, and burns.

It improves circulation and helps to soothe stiff and sore muscles.

It is great at healing congestion of the nose and killing illness caused by bugs in the air.

Among the conditions and illnesses alleviated by this oil are burns, blisters, cuts, herpes, insect bites, skin infections (including those caused by lice), and wounds. It also works as an insect repellent.

EUCALYPTUS, LEMON-SCENTED
Eucalyptus citriodora

The properties of this variety of eucalyptus are very similar to the previous one but it has a more pleasant smell.

FENNEL
Foeniculum vulgare

Fennel is known as a slimming herb. The essential oil is effective at reducing edema and promoting the removal of toxins. It will also help nursing mothers to produce more milk and can be useful in treating the symptoms of menopause.

A MUST-HAVE OIL

FRANKINCENSE
Boswellia carteri

Frankincense is most revered for its ability to soothe a troubled mind. It has long been used during meditation practices for this very reason. It is also very good for treating dry skin and reducing the appearance of wrinkle and scars.

It will help you overcome many respiratory-tract infections and can help to reduce the chances of an asthma attack.

GALBANUM
Ferula galbaniflua

Galbanum is useful in treating the skin. It helps improve skin tone and reduces the appearance of wrinkles and scars. It boosts circulation and helps to treat sore and stiff muscles. It alleviates coughs and has a strong antispasmodic effect. It also eases anxiety.

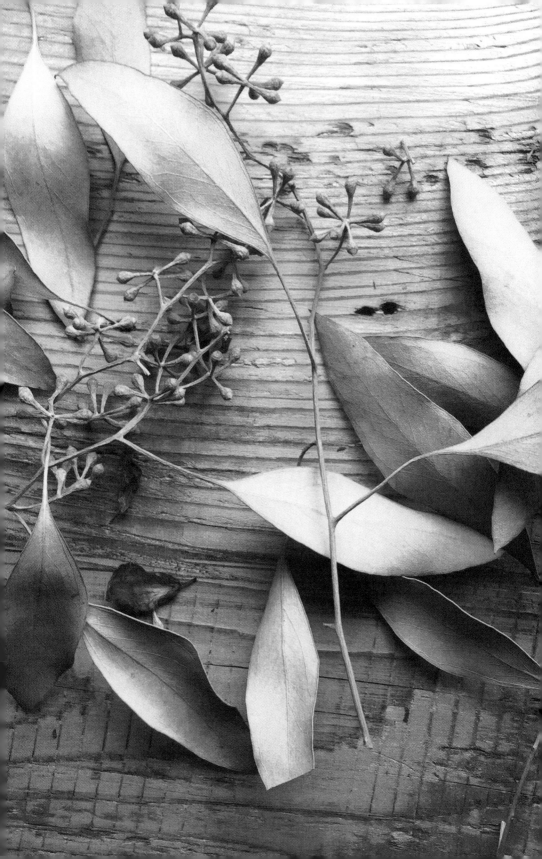

GERANIUM

Pelargonium graveolens

Geranium is one of the most useful oils when it comes to dealing with skin complaints. It helps heal everything from dermatitis to ringworm. It clears up the complexion and helps to rebalance the skin's sebum production.

It should not be used during the first trimester of pregnancy as it stimulates contractions of the uterus and so could cause a miscarriage.

GINGER

Zingiber officinale

Ginger is a warming oil and is very useful when it comes to muscular aches and pains. It boosts the circulation and helps to ease pain. It is useful in treating digestive upsets, infectious diseases, and colds and flu.

It also helps you overcome frailty related to stress.

GRAPEFRUIT

Citrus paradisi

This is useful in treating acne-prone and greasy skin. It helps to tone the skin and its underlying tissues, and revs up circulation. It stimulates the lymphatic system and eases water retention.

It has an energizing effect on the mind and can help with muscle fatigue as well.

GUAIACWOOD

Bulnesia sarmientoi

This is good for arthritis, gout, and rheumatism.

HELICHRYSUM

Helichrysum angustifolium

Helichrysum is another of the oils that is wonderful for the skin. It helps the skin heal and reduces inflammation. It is useful in treating stiff and sore muscles, as well as respiratory-tract infections.

HOPS

Humulus lupulus

Hops are best known for their soothing effect on the nervous system, but they are also useful in addressing problems with the menstrual cycle.

HYSSOP

Hyssopus officinalis

Hyssop is excellent for the skin and can help regulate blood pressure. It is useful in treating respiratory-tract infections and asthma.

A MUST-HAVE OIL

JASMINE

Jasminum officinale

Jasmine is most useful for the effect it has on the nervous system. It helps to build confidence and creates a euphoric sensation.

JUNIPER

Juniperus communis

Juniper oil is especially versatile if you want to detoxify your system or lose weight. It helps to tone the skin and is well suited to those with oily skin.

It helps to reduce anxiety and is useful in treating stiff and sore muscles.

LABDANUM

Cistus ladanifer

This is useful when you have mature skin and want to reduce the appearance of wrinkles.

A MUST-HAVE OIL

LAVENDER

Lavandula angustifolia

Lavender can be applied directly to the skin and has a wide range of uses. It will help to heal skin infections, fungal infections, allergic reactions, inflammation, and it also takes the sting out of burns.

It has antispasmodic and analgesic effects, making it a good treatment when you have sore muscles or joints. It works well alongside Tea Tree oil and Eucalyptus oil to reduce congestion and to alleviate colds and flu. It is a calming oil and can help you fall asleep more easily. It soothes anxiety caused by stress and is excellent at easing a headache.

A MUST-HAVE OIL

LEMON

Citrus limon

Lemon oil promotes circulation. It helps to strengthen nails and can normalize oily skin. It also helps to get rid of fever blisters. Lemon will normalize blood pressure and promote weight loss.

LEMON BALM

Melissa officinalis

Lemon balm is best known for its positive effect on the nervous system. It helps you overcome depression, anxiety, and insomnia, and helps treat cases of shock. For skin care, it is useful when it comes to treating problems like eczema.

A MUST-HAVE OIL

LEMONGRASS

Cymbopogon citratus

Lemongrass oil is a fantastic tissue toner and antifungal agent. It helps to improve circulation and muscle tone, and can ease stiff and sore muscles. It is an excellent remedy for trigger finger and texting thumb when applied topically to the affected area.

It is good at bringing down a fever and protecting against infectious diseases. It will also help to combat gastroenteritis. Lemongrass can give you a boost when you are too tired to think clearly.

LIME

Citrus aurantifolia

Lime is an uplifting oil that is great to use when you are under a lot of pressure. It is excellent for the skin and will help to open the pores; tone the tissues; and clear dull, dead skin. You should not expose the skin to the sun within an hour of applying the oil as it is phototoxic. This means that it will cause a reaction with the skin if you use it too soon before going out into the sun.

LINALOE

Bursera glabrifolia

Linaloe is useful for all skin types and is a great skin healer. It has a soothing effect on the nervous system.

LINDEN

Tilia vulgaris

This is best used for treating insomnia, headaches, and migraines, especially if these are brought on by stress.

LITSEA CUBEBA

Litsea cubeba

This is ideal for people who have oily skin or who suffer with excessive perspiration.

It is a valuable oil when it comes to sanitizing areas.

LOVAGE

Levisticum officinale

Lovage is excellent for detoxifying the body and reducing water retention. It boosts circulation and can normalize the menstrual cycle.

MANDARIN

Citrus reticulata

Mandarin oil is quite gentle and is suitable to use during pregnancy or on children older than two years. It is very useful for the skin—it clears dull skin and reduces the appearance of scars and stretch marks.

It is an excellent oil for soothing nervous tension and promoting a sound night's sleep.

MARIGOLD
Calendula officinalis

This oil is one of the most valuable skin healers. It soothes inflamed skin and promotes healing.

MARJORAM, SWEET
Origanum majorana

This oil is especially useful when it comes to easing stiff and sore muscles, anxiety, and insomnia.

MIMOSA
Acacia dealbata

Mimosa is good for people who have a tendency to overreact.

MYRRH
Commiphora myrrha

Myrrh is wonderful in treating mouth infections and ulcers. It also helps if you have dry skin or eczema.

MYRTLE
Myrtus communis

This is a good oil to use for children over the age of two because it is mild. It is valuable in the treatment of respiratory-tract ailments.

NEROLI

Citrus aurantium var. amara

Neroli is useful in clearing up dull skin and reducing the appearance of stretch marks and scars. It is an excellent oil to help lift the spirits and reduce anxiety.

NIAOULI

Melaleuca viridiflora

Niaouli is great for oily skin and helps clear up a number of skin conditions. It is very useful for treating respiratory-tract infections as well.

PALMAROSA

Cymbopogon martinii var. martinii

Palmarosa is one of the most valuable skin treatment options. It stimulates the regeneration of the skin, regulates the production of sebum, and moisturizes the tissue.

PATCHOULI

Pogostemon cablin

Patchouli is best known for its skin care properties. It is good for very dry skin and helps clear up fungal infections. It also helps regulate oil production in the skin and hair.

PARSLEY

Petroselinum sativum

Parsley oil is very useful for detoxifying your system. It also helps alleviate flatulence and clears up a urinary-tract infection.

A MUST-HAVE OIL

PEPPERMINT

Mentha piperita

Peppermint is most valuable as an aid to alertness and in clearing up colds and flu. Blended with eucalyptus, there is no better remedy for a blocked nose. Good for short-term use only. Isolated studies have linked long-term peppermint supplementation with Parkinson's Disease.

PERU BALSAM

Myroxylon balsamum var. pereirae

Peru balsam is a comforting oil to use during times of stress. It is an excellent balm for dry skin, sores, and rashes.

PETITGRAIN

Citrus aurantium var. amara

This is excellent for skin and hair that is greasy and also for curbing excessive perspiration.

PINE, LONGLEAF

Pinus palustris

Pine is extremely useful when it comes to respiratory-tract infections. It is also valuable in treating sore and stiff muscles and boosting circulation.

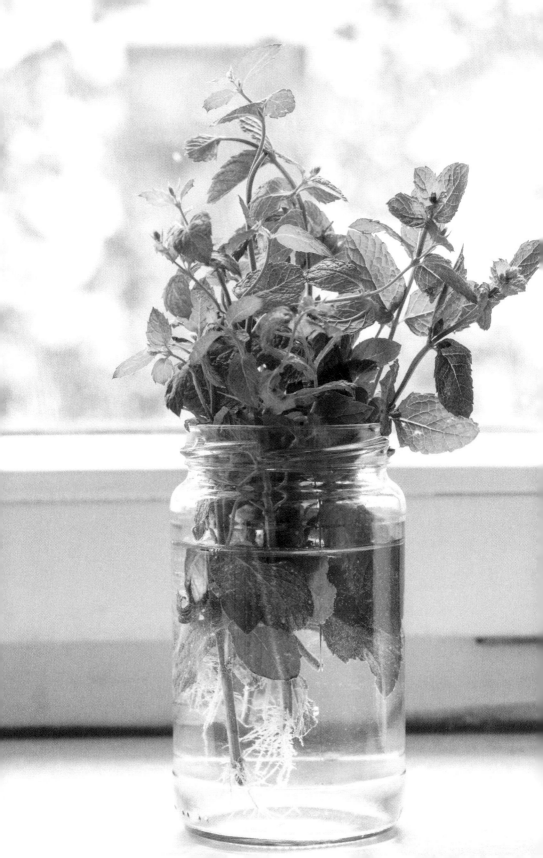

ROSE

Rosa centifolia

Rose oil is extremely useful for the skin and healing for dry, mature skin. It has a balancing effect on the female reproductive system. It is most useful for its ability to lift the emotions and instill a sense of optimism. People also feel it creates an air of romance and symbolizes devotion.

ROSEMARY

Rosmarinus officinalis

Rosemary is another oil that is excellent for promoting mental alertness. It is useful for treating oily skin and hair, and stimulates the growth of hair. It helps to reduce water retention and eases sore and stiff muscles. It boosts circulation.

SANDALWOOD

Santalum album

This is an oil that works well for dry or mature skin. It has a balancing effect on acne-prone or oily skin. It is extremely useful when it comes to anxiety-related stress and insomnia.

SPEARMINT

Mentha spicata

Spearmint is a lot gentler than peppermint and has similar properties. It helps to soothe digestive upsets and treat colds and flu.

SWEET ORANGE

Citrus sinensis

Sweet orange is great for dull complexions or oily skin. However, be sure not to use it just before going into the sun because it is phototoxic. It is also very useful for treating tension and depression.

A MUST-HAVE OIL

TEA TREE

Melaleuca alternifolia

Tea Tree oil can be applied directly to the skin. It has strong antibacterial, antiviral, and antifungal properties. Dilute it and use it sparingly unless it's thoroughly patch-tested.

A MUST-HAVE OIL

THYME

Thymus vulgaris

Thyme is very useful in combating infections of the respiratory tract. It will also help ease sore and stiff muscles, and improve circulation.

VALERIAN

Valeriana fauriei

Valerian is an oil that is best diffused. It helps to treat anxiety and stress, and will help you nod off at night.

VERBENA, LEMON

Aloysia triphylla

Lemon Verbena is most noted for its calming effect on the nervous system. It will also help you to get a good night's sleep.

VETIVER

Vetiveria zizanioides

Vetiver has several uses, but it is most valuable for its calming effect and the ability to quickly soothe tense and sore muscles.

YARROW

Achillea millefolium

Yarrow normalizes high blood pressure. It is useful in treating skin infections and reducing scarring. It will help you get over colds and flu, and reduces a fever.

A MUST-HAVE OIL

YLANG-YLANG

Cananga odorata var. genuina

Ylang-ylang has an exotic scent and is most prized for its ability to calm the mind and promote peaceful sleep. It is also a noted aphrodisiac oil.

That was quite a long list, wasn't it? Isn't it amazing what a few different plant essences can do? Now it's your turn to choose which one you are going to try.

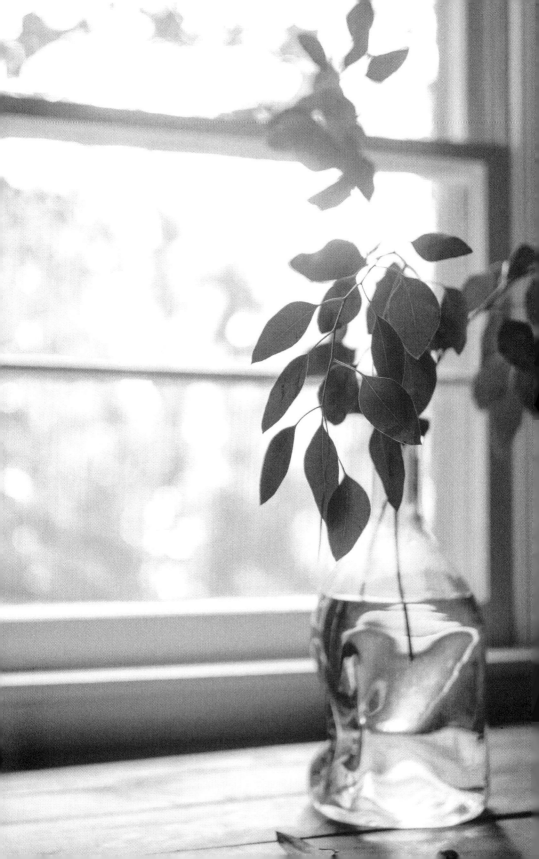

Chapter 5

Essential Oils for Weight Loss and Detoxification

M aintaining your ideal weight will give you a head start when it comes to being healthy. Now, when we are talking about being healthy here, we do not mean being stick-thin. Instead of worrying about being a set weight or size, you should use your body mass index (BMI) as a guide to whether or not you need to lose weight.

To figure out your BMI, you can easily Google "BMI Calculator" and input your height and weight. The system will then give you an estimated percentage of body fat.

* A BMI of less than 18.5 is considered underweight. If you fall into this category, you may want to consider trying to gain weight.

* A BMI of 18.5–24.9 is considered normal weight. If you fall into this category, you don't have to lose weight.

* A BMI of 25–29.9 is considered overweight. If you fall into this category, you may want to consider losing weight to enjoy more energy and better health.

* A BMI of 30 or above is considered obese. If you fall into this category, you need to lose weight to safeguard your health.

ESSENTIAL OILS AND DETOXIFICATION

When you're looking to detoxify, essential oils that are applied topically are of great benefit. (They must be diluted to a concentration of no more than 3 percent before being applied, though.) The oils are easily absorbed through the skin and into your bloodstream, meaning that they have a direct effect not only on the skin but on the circulation of the blood as well.

They stimulate the flow of lymph, helping to speed toxins out of your system. Lymphatic stimulants include lime, grapefruit, fennel, mandarin, white birch, and lemon.

ESSENTIAL OILS AND CIRCULATION

If you are looking for oils that boost circulation, and, subsequently, promote detoxification, look for oils that are classified as warming in nature. These oils not only speed the flow of blood to the area applied, they also influence the internal organs.

The upside of using warming oils is that many have analgesic properties. They help to reduce inflammation and numb the skin. They cause the blood vessels in the underlying tissues to expand, making it easier to move the blood in the area. This is crucial when it comes to bringing swelling down.

When the circulatory system is working as it should, your body becomes a lot more efficient and detoxification and weight loss become a lot easier.

Hyssop is a very useful essential oil if you have bad circulation. It has a balancing effect and will help to regulate your blood pressure as well.

Oils that help boost circulation include cypress, lemon, yarrow, and juniper.

BERGAMOT ESSENTIAL OIL

Citrus bergamia

Bergamot oil will improve your mood, relieve depression, and give you more energy.

Keep this on hand as an emergency treatment for times when you want to comfort yourself by eating or when you want to skip a workout. Bergamot helps you keep a sunny outlook. (Make sure to listen to your body and if you need to rest, do so! Lifelong health and vitality are a marathon not a sprint.)

BLACK PEPPER ESSENTIAL OIL

Piper nigrum

This is one of the spice oils and, as you might expect, it revs up circulation and your metabolism.

It has a strong analgesic and warming effect on sore and stiff muscles, arthritis, rheumatism, and the like. It can relieve neuralgia and improve muscle tone.

An antiviral and an antibiotic, Black Pepper essential oil is ideal for treating catarrh, colds, and flu.

It will help settle the stomach if rubbed into the abdomen and it is useful in treating bloating, diarrhea, constipation, and flatulence.

CINNAMON ESSENTIAL OIL

Cinnamomum zeylanicum

Cinnamon has been proven to regulate blood sugar, much as conventional medicines like Metformin do. By including half a teaspoon to a teaspoon of powdered cinnamon a day into your diet, you will see similar effects to what you would have had you been on medication to lower your blood sugar.

You can use the oil in a diffuser to help reduce cravings for sweets. This oil can irritate the skin, so if you apply it topically, you should always dilute it to around about 1 percent concentration.

The oil will also help to soothe digestive upsets and spasms within the digestive tract. This can be extremely useful when you first start a new diet, especially if the diet includes a lot of fiber.

This should not be used during pregnancy, as it stimulates contractions of the uterus and so could cause a miscarriage.

Cinnamon can give you a nice boost when you are feeling down and exhausted due to stress.

The very scent of cinnamon creates a feeling of nostalgia by reminding you of holiday times and all those great feelings. It instills in you a feeling that you can handle just about anything.

EUCALYPTUS ESSENTIAL OIL
Eucalyptus globules

Eucalyptus oil is extremely useful to have on hand, especially if you have started a new exercise regimen to help you lose weight. It helps to rev up the circulation and can be used in a muscle rub to reduce stiffness and swelling.

If you suffer from rheumatoid arthritis, sprains, or similar aches and pains, eucalyptus should be on your list. It is a great oil to get you back on your feet when you have a respiratory-tract infection. It will help clear up congestion and neutralize airborne infectious agents.

Eucalyptus oil can help relieve headaches as well. It has a clear, clean scent that can also be useful to get rid of lethargy.

FENNEL ESSENTIAL OIL
Foeniculum vulgare

Fennel has long been associated with weight loss because it has strong diuretic properties. The oil, when properly diluted, is very useful when it comes to losing water weight. It stimulates the lymphatic system and helps the tissues to speed excess water out of them.

Rub it into the abdomen to assist in treating dyspepsia, constipation, flatulence, and nausea.

Fennel has a delicate licorice scent that is soothing. It also has analgesic properties that make it useful in the treatment of rheumatism.

Ailments related to poor circulation like cellulitis and cellulite respond well to daily massages of Fennel oil.

GINGER ESSENTIAL OIL

Zingiber officinale

Ginger oil will help you when your get up and go has left. It helps to stimulate circulation and speed the removal of toxins from the blood. It helps to relieve sore and stiff muscles and gives you a boost of energy when you are fatigued.

It is warming and when rubbed into the skin will boost the circulation in the area and gently warm it. It is useful for treating sprained and strained muscles as well.

You can rub diluted Ginger oil onto your abdomen to help reduce indigestion, flatulence, cramps, and diarrhea.

It helps to get rid of colds and flu and, if diffused, helps to protect against airborne infectious microbes.

If you need a hit of energy, Ginger oil will give you the boost that you need.

GRAPEFRUIT ESSENTIAL OIL

Citrus paradisi

Grapefruit and grapefruit extract have long been linked with weight loss. If you cannot handle the sour taste of the fruit, you can get some of the benefits by using Grapefruit essential oil. The oil should be diluted and applied topically, added to the bath, or diffused.

Grapefruit essential oil is phototoxic. The skin could become irritated, darkened, or even burned. To avoid this, wait at least an hour before exposing yourself to UV radiation.

The oil will help rev up your system, give you energy, and stimulate circulation. Mix a handful of sea salt, 2 drops of oil, and enough olive oil to form a paste and use as a body scrub.

Grapefruit oil will help you overcome stress and fatigue, and also help boost your metabolism.

JUNIPER ESSENTIAL OIL

Juniperus communis

This is one of the top oils to use if you want to lose weight. The scent is pleasant and the oil will give your circulatory system a good kick start. Mix with equal parts of Sweet Orange essential oil and Eucalyptus essential oil and a carrier oil. Rub the mixture onto your body just before you take a hot bath to boost circulation and help remove toxins from the bloodstream.

Juniper oil helps to reduce anxiety and tension, and will help you get over colds and flu as well.

LEMON ESSENTIAL OIL

Citrus limon

Lemon essential oil is a citrus oil that has a similar effect to Grapefruit oil. It has a wonderful clean, energizing scent that is great first thing in the morning.

Rubbed into the skin in a suitable carrier oil, it will help to stimulate circulation and ease stiff and sore muscles. Lemon lifts the spirits and helps you keep your eye on the prize.

It is a phototoxic oil, so steer clear of UV radiation if you have applied it to your skin.

Fortunately, it is just as effective for lifting your mood when you diffuse it.

LEMONGRASS ESSENTIAL OIL

Cymbopogon citratus

We are mostly used to adding lemongrass to our food for the flavor it imparts. Lemongrass can be a lot more useful, though.

It assists in reducing muscle aches and pains and also helps to tone the muscles. It is wonderful for revving up your circulation.

It has strong antiviral and antibacterial properties, so it can help reduce the symptoms of colds and flu.

When rubbed into the abdomen, Lemongrass oil helps to treat indigestion and gastroenteritis.

If you are at your wit's end, this is a good oil to have on standby.

MANDARIN ESSENTIAL OIL

Citrus reticulata

Mandarin essential oil is gentler than other citrus oils, such as grapefruit and lemon. It is, however, very useful if you want to lose weight.

Apply the oil diluted in 1 teaspoon of Sweet Almond oil to help reduce the appearance of stretch marks and to prevent the formation of new stretch marks.

The oil calms an upset tummy and is very soothing in response to nervous tension as well.

The oil is phototoxic, so it shouldn't be applied directly before exposure to the sun.

The oil is safe to use during pregnancy.

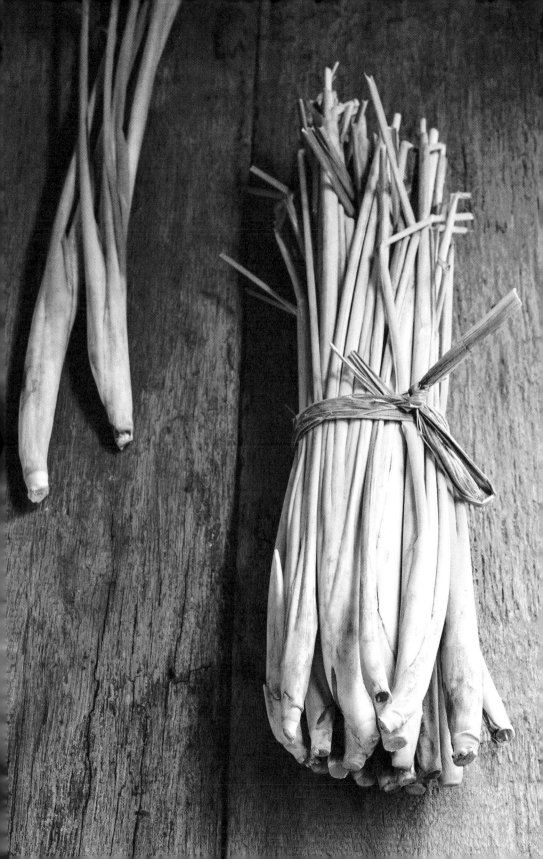

PEPPERMINT ESSENTIAL OIL

Mentha piperita

Peppermint essential oil is one of the best antispasmodic essential oils. It can irritate the skin, though, so be sure to dilute it well if you are applying it topically.

The oil helps to clear bloating and relieve dyspepsia.

You can also choose to diffuse it to help you improve your focus and increase alertness. Do not use it too close to bedtime or you might have trouble falling asleep.

Recipes to Help You Increase Your Fitness Level

Using the above-mentioned essential oils will help you to lose weight naturally. Here are some recipes that you can try for yourself.

DETOXIFYING BATH

Yields 1 bath

This recipe will allow you to have a bath that will likely be the most relaxing that you have ever had. That said, if you have high blood pressure, epilepsy, or are pregnant, you should not use this recipe at all. Keep a glass of water next to the bath and sip it throughout.

   1–2 cups Epsom salt

   ½ cup baking soda

   2 drops Sweet Orange oil

   2 drops Juniper oil

Draw the bath and keep it as hot as you can handle. Dissolve the Epsom salt and the baking soda into it. Add the oils just before you are ready to climb in. Soak in the bath for at least 25 minutes or so. When you get out, wrap yourself in a warm towel.

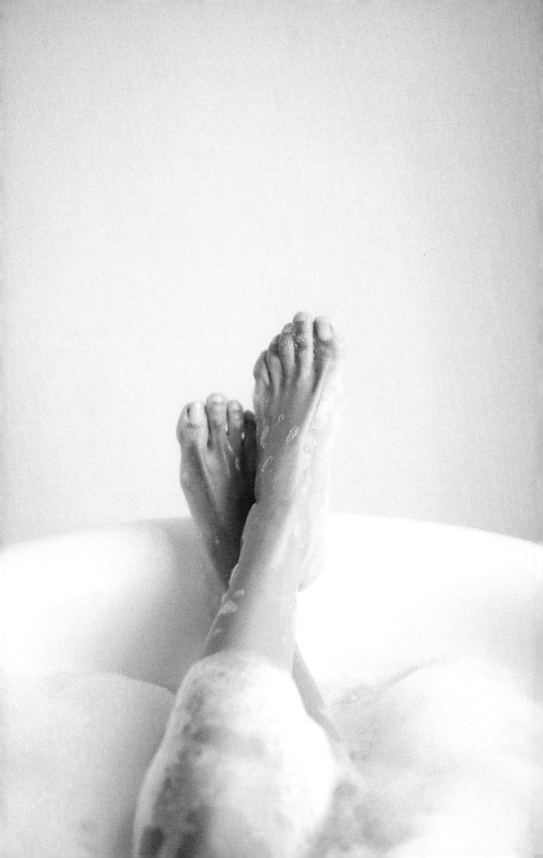

TONING SCRUB

Yields 2 cups

This recipe will invigorate your senses with its stimulating scent. The fennel is especially good to massage on your abdomen to relieve bloating. Let your muscles feel toned and rejuvenated with this delicious scrub.

> 1 cup coffee grounds
>
> 1 cup sea salt
>
> 5 drops Fennel oil
>
> 5 drops Grapefruit oil
>
> 5 drops Lemon oil

Blend all the ingredients and rub into the skin to exfoliate. Leave in place for a couple of minutes and rinse in the shower. If there is any mixture left over, store it for up to two days in an airtight container.

EXERCISE READINESS BLEND

Yields 4 ounces

Massage this peppery blend into your muscles before or after working out to increase energy and stamina. It will help you build your endurance and enjoy your workout!

> 100 ml Sweet Almond oil
>
> 5 drops Eucalyptus oil
>
> 5 drops Black Pepper oil
>
> 5 drops Grapefruit oil

Mix together and rub into sore, stiff muscles.

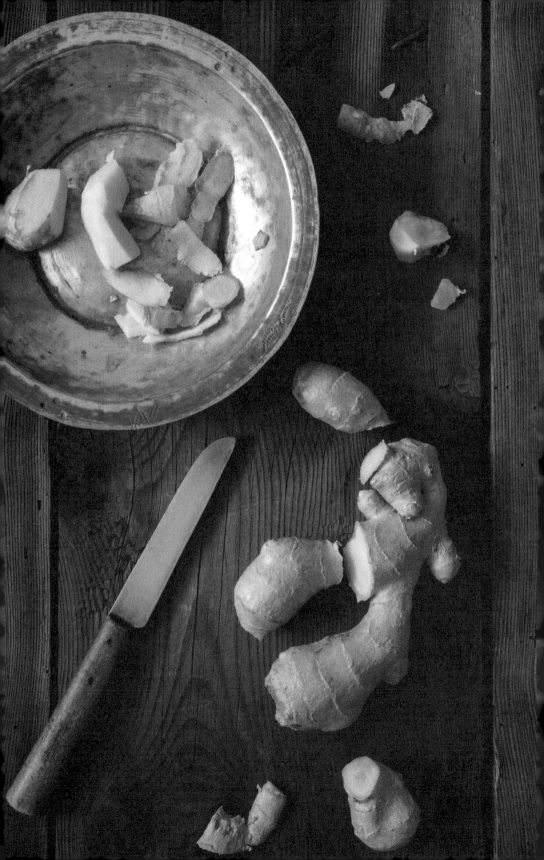

WAKE-ME-UP BLEND

Yields less than an ounce

Diffuse this warming and stimulating blend to enliven your environment. It is great to diffuse during the mid afternoon when some people feel an afternoon slump. Teachers can use this if the classroom requires more energy and participation from students.

    5 drops Ginger oil
    5 drops Grapefruit oil

Blend these oils and diffuse the mixture first thing in the morning to get you ready for the day.

CIRCULATION-STIMULATING OIL

Yields 4 ounces

Massage this blend into limbs and abdomen for a revivifying burst of warmth. This is especially useful during the colder months of the year. Let it fill your senses with sweet warmth and vitality.

    100 ml Sweet Almond oil
    5 drops Cinnamon oil
    5 drops Ginger oil

Mix together and apply topically.

*

You are now ready to go out and enjoy the benefits of essential oils on your own fitness and health journey.

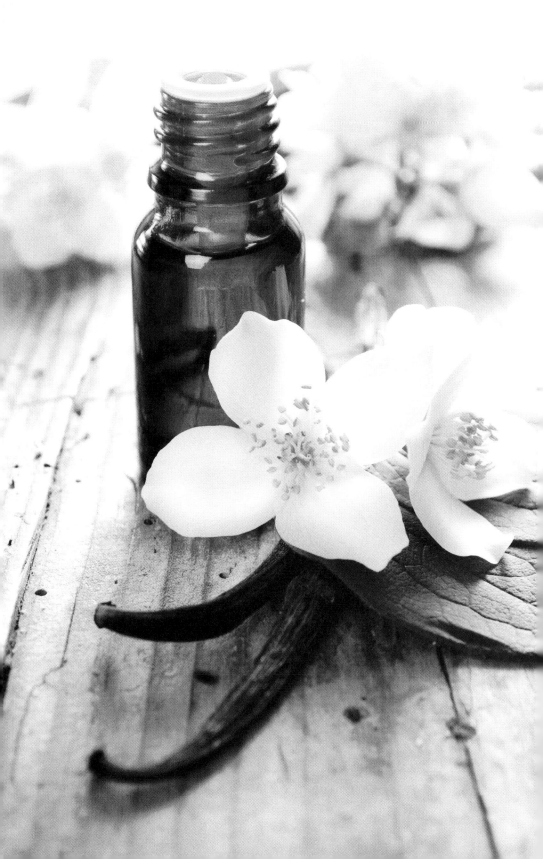

Chapter 6

Essential Oils for Skin, Hair, and Perfume

The skin is the largest organ in the human body and plays an extremely important role in our overall health and well-being—it protects our bodies from dangers in the outside world. The skin helps to keep out dangerous bacteria, regulate body temperature, repel water, and maintain the moisture balance our bodies require.

When we have skin and hair problems, this often points to a deeper problem, like higher toxicity levels, imbalances in the hormonal systems, or emotional issues. Essential oils are ideal for addressing both the symptoms and any underlying issues because they work on so many levels.

In this chapter, we will go through the best essential oils to keep your skin and hair in tip-top condition. We'll also have a quick look at what else the oils are good for. Finally, we'll wrap up with recipes that you can try out for yourself.

Before we start, though, keep in mind that none of the essential oils listed below should be used undiluted on the skin. They should always be diluted at a concentration of no more than 3 percent with a carrier oil or an aqueous cream. If you plan to use the blend on your face, be sure to decrease the concentration of oils.

BERGAMOT

Citrus bergamia

Bergamot oil is classified as a citrus oil, even though it has more of a floral scent. This oil is also phototoxic, so be sure not to come in contact with UV radiation within the first hour or so after application of the oil.

It is effective as an antibacterial agent and has astringent qualities, making it ideal for treating skin that is oily or acne-prone. It has a balancing effect in response to problem skin conditions, such as eczema.

It will help to relieve the itch of insect bites and eczema, and reduce the appearance of varicose veins and dark spots.

Add a few drops to your mouthwash to help treat bad breath and mouth ulcers.

You can also make up a cream or douche to help clear up vaginal discharge.

The diluted oil may be applied to cold sores to help get rid of them.

CEDARWOOD, ATLAS

Cedrus atlantica

Cedarwood oil has a deep, earthy scent. It is a woody oil, like Sandalwood, but it's more astringent. It should be used by people who have oily skin, rather than those with dry skin. It helps in the treatment of acne, eczema, dermatitis, and pimples.

If you have problems with dandruff, a few drops of this oil, mixed into a base of Sweet Almond oil and rubbed into the scalp regularly will help to relieve the symptoms. It will also help prevent hair loss.

Because it has a strong antifungal action, Cedarwood oil can be used to treat conditions such as ringworm and thrush. It is useful in the treatment of vaginal discharge. It also alleviates stress-related conditions.

GERANIUM

Pelargonium graveolens

Geranium oil is often used as a substitute for Rose oil because they have similar benefits. The scent of Geranium oil may be overpowering, however. If that bothers you, use only 1 drop of Geranium oil for every 2 drops of other oils. Despite the strong scent, if you only want to get one oil on this list, this should be it.

Geranium's primary benefit is in its ability to treat various skin conditions. No other oil even comes close. It can be used by all skin types and will help to balance the sebum levels of the skin. If you have acne-prone skin, applying Geranium oil will help to reduce the severity of breakouts, ease inflammation, and prevent infections and scarring. It promotes regeneration of the skin, so it is excellent to use for reducing the appearance of scars.

It is anti-inflammatory and soothes skin that is irritated or inflamed. It does a great job in the treatment of eczema. It has antihistaminic properties, so it can be used to treat allergic skin reactions. It will reduce the inflammation and soothe itching as well.

It also has analgesic properties; as a result, it can be applied to sore, burned skin to help relieve pain and promote healing.

Geranium oil also helps to boost circulation. Create a salt rub by mixing 3 tablespoons sea salt with a few drops of Geranium and Juniper oil. Mix in enough olive oil to create a paste and rub it into areas that are rough or where you have cellulite. Rinse it off in the shower. Your skin will be softer and smoother, and your circulation will be boosted.

If your skin problems are related to hormonal upsets, Geranium oil should be on your list. It helps to gently rebalance the hormonal system. Because of this effect, though, women who have been diagnosed with ovarian or breast cancer should not use this oil.

It should also be avoided during the first trimester of pregnancy.

If your skin problems are due to stress or depression, Geranium oil should be considered. It helps to rebalance the emotions, lift your mood, and induce relaxation.

JASMINE
Jasminum officinale

It takes upwards of 3.5 million petals to make about a pound of Jasmine absolute, and this makes the oil extremely expensive. Most of what you find in the stores is jasmine blended with other oils.

Fortunately, a little bit of jasmine goes a long way and, as long as you choose a reputable brand of blended oil, you can still reap the benefits.

Jasmine is wonderful for the skin and for creating a feeling of contentment. If your skin problems stem from an emotional upheaval or another source of depression, jasmine will soothe both the skin and the mind.

JUNIPER
Juniperus communis

Juniper oil is one of the oils best suited to oily skin, rather than dry skin. It is astringent and clarifies the skin. It is useful in the treatment of acne. It also helps alleviate problematic skin conditions, such as dermatitis and eczema.

A blend of equal parts of Juniper and Cedarwood oils, mixed with a carrier oil and massaged into the scalp, can help to prevent hair loss.

Juniper oil helps to stimulate the lymphatic system and is effective at clearing out toxins and boosting circulation. This makes it useful in treating cellulite and promoting weight loss

The oil has a clearing and uplifting effect on the mind as well.

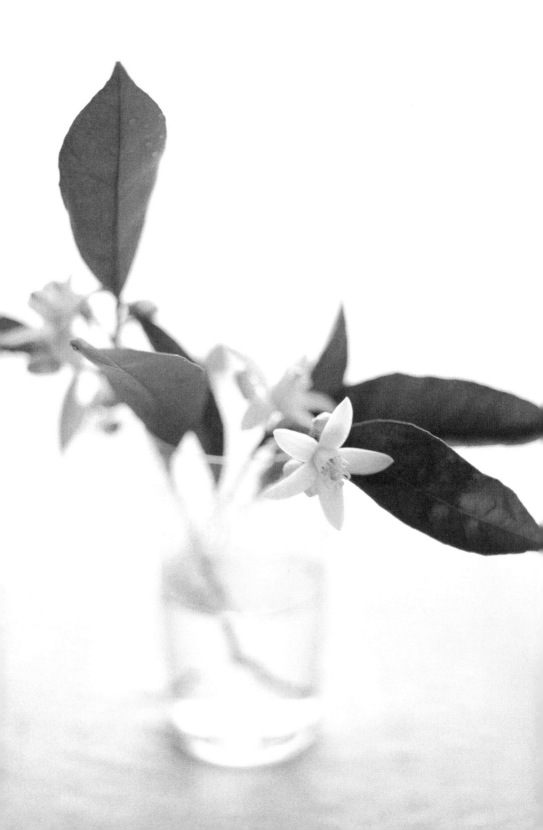

NEROLI

Citrus aurantium var. amara

Neroli is an especially wonderful scented oil. It will blend with most other oils and does a great job lifting your mood and balancing the emotions.

When using Neroli oil, though, you need to be aware that it is phototoxic. That means that if you are exposed to UV light, such as from the sun or a tanning bed, too soon after applying the oil, it will cause a reaction. This could result in darkening of or damage to the skin, or heightened skin sensitivity and irritation. The phototoxicity issue need not be a major one—simply apply the oil only at night or at least an hour before you go out into the sun.

Neroli is ideal if you have very dry, dull, or sensitive skin. It is also excellent at promoting the turnover of skin cells and useful when it comes to reducing the appearance of scars.

Blending 3 drops of Geranium oil and half a cup of Rose Hip oil and adding 5 drops of Neroli oil makes a scar treatment that is hard to beat.

Blended with 3 drops of Sandalwood oil, a small amount of Avocado oil and Sweet Almond oil, it will help to restore the skin's natural sebum function and prevent dullness and dryness.

If you have problems with circulation, neroli can be tonifying and fortifying.

Neroli, Palmarosa, and Geranium oils, mixed in equal parts and diluted with a good-quality aqueous cream, make an outstanding treatment for eczema.

Cymbopogon martinii var. martini

Palmarosa is your skin's friend. Because it stimulates cellular regeneration, it is helpful in the prevention of wrinkles and in the treatment of scars.

It helps to regulate sebum production and to treat both dry skin and acne.

Its antibacterial properties make it useful in treating minor cuts, scrapes, and infections.

It also helps to soothe dermatitis and reduce the irritation related to it.

It can address nervous exhaustion and ease stress-related conditions.

ROSE

Rosa centifolia

Pure Rose Otto oil is only extracted from the petals of the rose, as opposed to many parts of the plant, so, like jasmine, it is very expensive to produce. Again, most of what you find in stores will be a blended oil. Again, a little bit of Rose oil goes a long way.

The name rose otto signifies that the oil from the rose was extracted using a gentler, steam-based method than that used in making Rose absolute oil, which is extracted using a solvent method (see page 14).

Choosing a quality brand of the blended oil gives you the best of both worlds—an affordable price and a good therapeutic product. Five drops of both Rose and Jasmine oils blended together leave the skin deliciously scented and can form the basis for a lovely perfume.

Rose is a wonderful oil to use during times of stress and when you are feeling low. It helps to balance the emotions and induce relaxation.

As an ally for the skin, it is hard to beat Rose oil. It soothes and heals burned or irritated skin, and promotes the regeneration of the tissue. It minimizes the appearance of thread veins and fine lines. It is especially good for skin that is very dry or sensitive.

SANDALWOOD

Santalum album

If you are planning to make your own perfumes, Sandalwood oil is a must to have on hand. It is excellent as a fixative. In other words, it grounds the scents of the more volatile oils, such as Jasmine oil, and helps the blend retain its scent for a longer time.

If you have very dry skin, this is one of the best oils you can use. Make a blend of equal parts of Sandalwood, Palmarosa, Geranium, and Neroli oils, and mix the blend into a good-quality aqueous base for a wonderful night cream.

If you are going through a tough time, or are battling to relax and get enough sleep, Sandalwood oil will help to induce relaxation and promote deeper sleep.

YLANG-YLANG

Cananga odorata var. genuina

Of all the essential oils, this one smells the most exotic. It is also one of the only oils that has a completely balanced scent and can be used on its own as a perfume. Because of the heady scent of this oil, it is important to use it sparingly—a little goes a long way. If used in too high a concentration, it can bring on or worsen a headache.

It is especially useful in balancing the sebum levels in your skin. It is appropriate for all skin types.

Try adding a few drops into the rinse water when washing your hair to increase shine and leave a delicate scent.

Ylang-ylang is a deeply relaxing essential oil and renowned for its prowess as an aphrodisiac. It helps to relax the body and mind, and can be useful in helping you to nod off to sleep. Again, use only a drop or two on your pillow or the scent could be overwhelming.

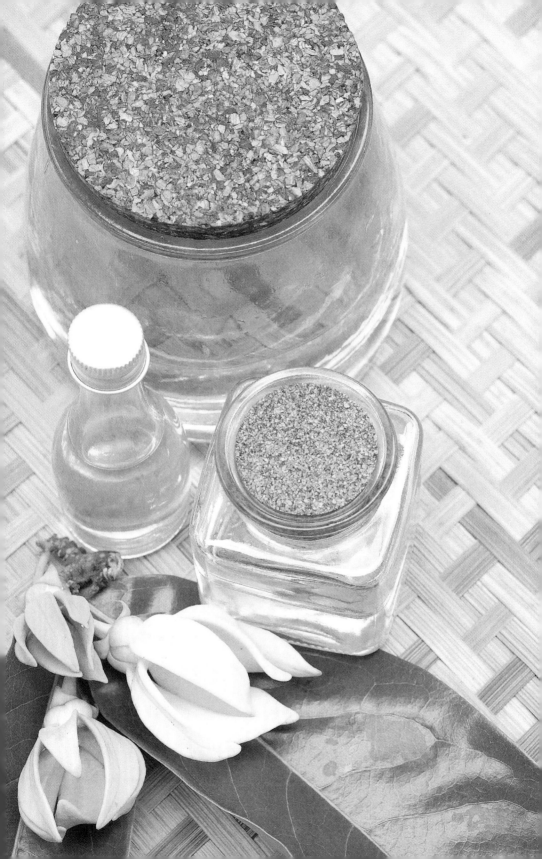

Radiant Skin and Hair Recipes

ANTI-MITE SHAMPOO

This recipe is useful in treating Demodex mite overgrowth. We all have Demodex mites on our skin; in some adults, these organisms cause an overgrowth and infestation on the eyelashes or other parts of the body where hair grows. Demodex mites are also implicated as a potential cause of rosacea. The good news is that Tea Tree oil can reduce any infestation easily and naturally. So you can use this shampoo as a preventive several times a month or whenever you feel the need.

    2–4 tablespoons organic shampoo
    1–3 drops Tea Tree oil

Place the shampoo in the palm of your hand and then drop a couple drops of Tea Tree oil in and mix it in your palm. Massage into your scalp for several minutes and be sure to not allow this mixture to run into your eyes.

DRY SHAMPOO

If you are pressed for time and don't have time for a shower or your hair is color treated or dry and you don't want to wash it every time you shower, this recipe is for you! Use this delightful smelling dry shampoo to mop up excess oil at the scalp and leave your hair smelling delicious. Bonus if you highlight your hair and have dark roots growing in, this mixture will lighten them up a bit!

    1 drop Cedarwood oil
    1 tablespoon cornstarch or powdered orris root

Mix ingredients well and then rub gently into the oily areas on your scalp. Let it sit for a few minutes before brushing it out.

DRY SKIN SERUM

If your skin tends to be on the dry side you can use this feminine and lovely smelling blend to moisturize and add vital rejuvenation to your complexion. It minimizes fine lines and promotes collagen production.

    100 ml Rose Hip oil
    5 drops Rose oil
    5 drops Neroli oil

Pat onto your face just after cleansing. Let it sink in for at least five minutes and then pat off excess with a tissue. Follow with your normal moisturizer, if you like. Rose Hip oil has antioxidant properties because of the plant's high vitamin C content.

GOOD MORNING LOTION

Say good morning to your skin with this enchanting treat. The mixture is fortifying from the Sandalwood and tonifying via the slightly astringent quality of the Geranium. Add in some exotic Palmarosa and you have the recipe for a day that is sunny side up.

> 500 ml aqueous cream or unscented body lotion
>
> 10 drops Sandalwood oil
>
> 5 drops Geranium oil
>
> 10 drops Palmarosa oil

Mix everything together well. There are no phototoxic ingredients in this lotion so you can apply it morning or evening.

HAIR TONIC

Make your hair extra shiny with this brightening rinse. The apple cider vinegar balances the hair's Ph and lets your hair's natural luster shine through. Meanwhile, the geranium or sandalwood minimize oiliness while the lavender and rose water both add a delightful scent.

> 10 drops Geranium or Sandalwood oil (depending on whether your hair is dry or not)
>
> 1 tablespoon apple cider vinegar
>
> 100 ml Lavender oil or Rose Water

Mix everything together and massage into your scalp. If possible, let it stay there overnight or as long as possible before rinsing your hair.

HEAVENLY BODY LOTION

This lotion is a little slice of heaven. It will fill your senses with aromas both exotic and relaxing. It's the perfect recipe for reducing stress and having a pleasant and productive evening.

 450 ml aqueous cream or unscented body lotion of your choice

 10 drops Sandalwood oil

 50 ml Rose Hip oil

 10 drops Neroli oil

 10 drops Rose oil

 10 drops Palmarosa oil

Mix everything together well. This should be applied after your shower at night and only at night because of the photosensitivity of the Neroli oil. This blend smells great and is very relaxing.

SCALP RUB

This divinely scented blend will reduce dry scalp and soothe scaliness. The Cedarwood and Coconut promote healthy hair growth. The juniper stimulates the hair follicles with its gentle astringent nature.

 5 drops Cedarwood oil

 5 drops Juniper oil

 100 ml Coconut Oil

Mix together all the ingredients. Massage a small amount into your scalp about half an hour before you shower. In the shower, mix your shampoo with a little bit of warm water and massage into the scalp. Then rinse everything out.

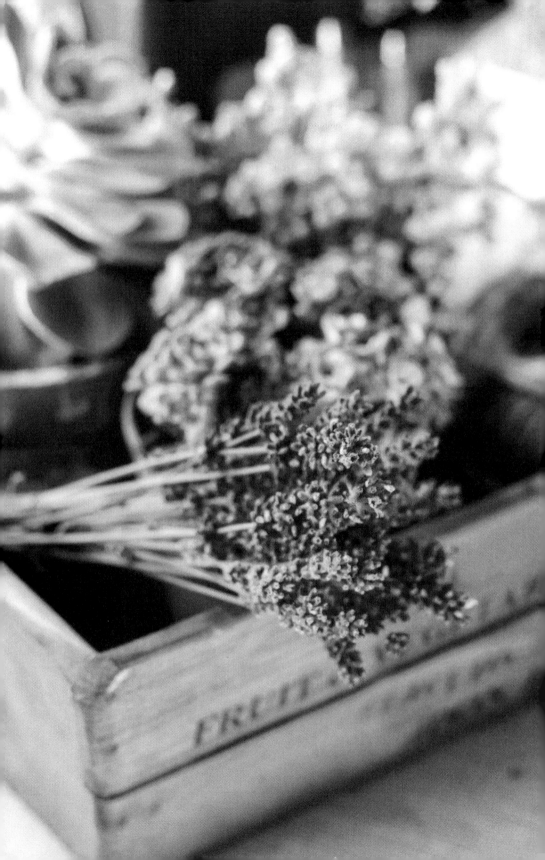

Chapter 7

Essential Oils for the Home

We do a lot to keep ourselves healthy and safe—we make sure that our homes are sanitized, protect ourselves against bugs, and take care of all the minor scrapes and sniffles along the way. We have pills to take when we are sick, a whole range of cleaning products to use, and even sprays to keep bugs at bay.

If you think of all the products that we have at our disposal, you'd think that we'd all be healthy and happy. But those very chemicals that we use to keep ourselves safe are actually slowly destroying our health.

Take *xenoestrogens*, for example. These are a type of endocrine disruptor that mimics estrogen in the body. What that means is that they have a massive impact on normal hormone function, leaving you at risk of developing signs of estrogen dominance.

If left unchecked, estrogen dominance has very serious deleterious effects on your health. It increases the risk of infertility, obesity, breast cancer, endometriosis, diabetes, and miscarriage. In young girls, it can cause early-onset puberty. And men are also not immune to its effects—it increases the chances of a man developing testicular cancer and prostate cancer.

Here's an alarming fact—you are being exposed to xenoestrogens every day. They are present in many of the products that you use on a daily basis.

HOW TO LIMIT YOUR EXPOSURE

The best way to limit your exposure to chemicals is to start changing the products you use every day. Cutting back on your use of plastic and human-made chemicals as much as possible is the best thing you can do for your health today.

And the good news is that this is actually going to be a lot easier than you think. You can rely on Mother Nature to provide a natural solution for you that is not only just as effective as the chemicals, but also great for your health.

Essential oils are made up of a number of powerful natural compounds. These compounds have been designed by nature to help plants thrive and ward off disease. They can do the same for you.

All essential oils have some kind of antibacterial properties, so they can be incorporated into your home-cleaning routine. Studies show that Eucalyptus oil, for example, is as powerful an antibacterial agent as many common cleaning compounds, without the negative side effects.

Essential oils can be used as a part of your first aid kit as well. They can reduce pain, fight infections, and promote healing. And they smell great, too. There are many practical applications for essential oils. For example, citronella repels bugs.

Let's examine the essential oils that you should consider incorporating in your first-aid, insect-repelling, and cleaning routines. We'll go through what the benefits of each oil are and then wrap up with some great recipes for you to make. Before we start, though, unless otherwise stated, keep in mind that essential oils should never be applied directly to the skin—most must be mixed with a carrier oil or an aqueous cream at a concentration of no more than 3 percent before being applied topically.

It doesn't get much greener than essential oils: when used correctly, they are among Mother Nature's most potent remedies.

BASIL

Ocimum basilicum

One of the "kitchen" herbs, Basil oil also has an extremely strong smell. It is also one of the best oils to have on hand when you really need to focus. You can make the scent a little less potent by mixing in Lime oil and Bergamot oil.

Basil oil helps to clear up a head cold in next to no time, and can help to clear the air of germs that cause colds and flu when diffused through the home or office.

It has a balancing effect on the mind, making it ideal when you are feeling stressed or anxious.

A Basil oil blend, when rubbed onto the abdomen, will help to relieve an upset stomach and cramping related to menstruation. When rubbed into sore muscles, it brings relief quickly.

Basil oil can be used during your cleaning routine to help disinfect the home.

It acts as a strong insect repellent, especially when combined with Citronella oil.

If you are pregnant, you should not use Basil oil at all because it is too strong for your constitution at that time and may cause disruption to your system. In rare cases it could cause cramping.

When applying the oil topically, keep it at a low concentration (about 1 percent), as it may irritate the skin.

CHAMOMILE

Matricaria recutita

Chamomile, another extremely useful oil, is gentle and can be used on kids age 10 weeks and older. It should be used diluted.

This has the best analgesic properties of all the oils. Blended with Lavender oil and diluted, it works wonders for a headache. It is also one of the best options when you have a bad toothache. Apply it to the cheek outside where the tooth is sore. Do not use it inside the mouth.

If you have an earache, a lavender and chamomile blend will soothe it.

Chamomile is also a good anti-inflammatory. Use it to help sore and stiff muscles and joints and for menstrual cramping. It will also soothe allergic skin conditions and eczema.

If you battle with insomnia or are stressed out, chamomile should be in your first aid kit. Boost its relaxing qualities by blending it with Lavender oil.

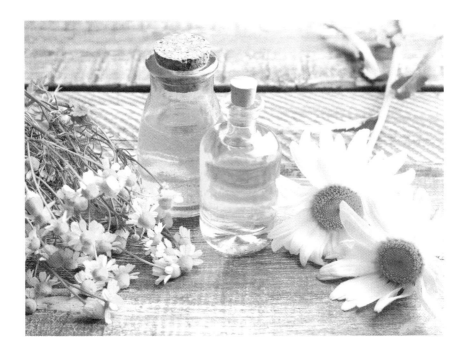

CITRONELLA

Cymbopogon nardus

Citronella oil is probably best known as a bug repellent, but there is a lot more to this oil as well.

It works well to clear up colds and flu and is a good oil to use to wake you up.

In addition, Citronella oil helps with headaches, neuralgia, and migraines.

EUCALYPTUS

Eucalyptus globulus

This is an extremely useful oil. It should not, however, be applied directly on the skin. Either add a few drops to your bath, diffuse the oil, or add it to a carrier oil when applying it directly to the skin.

Eucalyptus has a strong, clean smell and potent antiviral and antibacterial properties. It will help to clear up congested sinuses and combat the symptoms of colds and flu. It will also help keep viruses from spreading.

This oil is particularly good for soothing aching muscles after hitting the gym hard.

Mix it into the rinse water when wiping down your counters to disinfect them and keep flies at bay.

LAVENDER

Lavandula angustifolia

Most people will recognize this oil. It is one of the best loved and most recognizable of all the essential oils. It is also one of the most useful. If you just get one bottle of essential oil, this should be it.

Lavender oil is one of the only oils that can be applied directly to your skin. It is even safe to use on children from the age of 10 weeks on up. Keep lavender oil on hand to treat burns, minor cuts, scrapes, scratches, insect bites, and bruises. It is a good analgesic and can be topically applied to reduce pain. It will soothe inflammation and also help to calm allergic reactions. In addition, because it is a strong antifungal agent, it can be applied right to fungal infections, such as ringworm.

It is a wonderful skin healer, promoting skin regeneration and preventing scarring. It can be used in a diffuser to decongest the sinuses or help to soothe a bad cough. It is also extremely useful if you have a headache or are trying to sleep. Either use it in a diffuser or rub a drop or two into each temple for fast relief.

Add a few drops to your bathwater or mix it into your favorite body lotion to help soothe aching muscles.

PEPPERMINT

Mentha piperita

Peppermint is another of those broadly useful oils that should be a staple in your home.

It works extremely well to help decongest the sinuses and fight colds and flu, and helps to soothe and warm stiff and sore muscles. To boost these effects, blend Peppermint and Eucalyptus oils.

If you have indigestion, bloating, or flatulence, a Peppermint oil blend can be very helpful.

Be careful not to use the oil too late at night, as it stimulates the mind and might keep you awake.

If you are on a homeopathic medicine regimen, or are pregnant, do not use Peppermint oil because it is too stimulating for pregnant women and there have not been enough studies to confirm its safety. Best for only short-term use when taken internally.

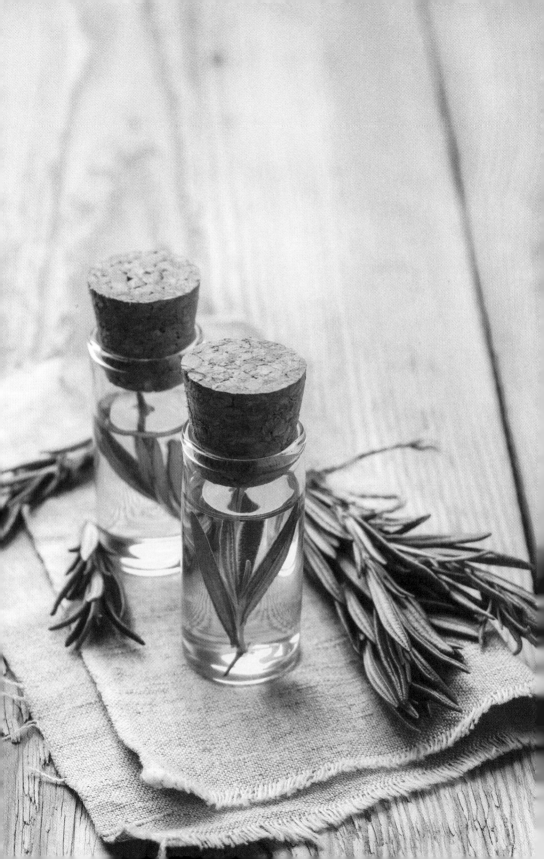

ROSEMARY

Rosmarinus officinalis

You are either going to love it or hate it. Rosemary has a strong scent that can quickly overpower a blend. For this reason, use half as much Rosemary oil as you do your other oils.

Rosemary is best known for its ability to clear foggy thinking and help you to stay alert. Roman soldiers used to place a sprig of rosemary behind their ears before going into battle to sharpen their reflexes.

If you have a long night ahead, a few drops each of Rosemary and Peppermint oils on a tissue that you sniff regularly will help you stay awake. It will also help ease an upset stomach and promote detoxification when a couple drops of these two oils are rubbed onto the abdomen.

Rosemary oil helps to treat respiratory-tract infections. Blended with Eucalyptus oil, it makes a potent antiviral agent.

If you have a headache brought on by stress, apply a blend of 1 drop of Rosemary and three drops of Lavender oils to the temples. Alternatively, add this blend to water, make a cold compress, and apply it that way.

Rosemary stimulates your circulation and helps to soothe aching muscles.

Rosemary should not be used by women who are pregnant. It has powerful properties that may be too astringent and overpowering for your baby.

SWEET MARJORAM

Origanum majorana

This is a strongly scented oil, but don't let that put you off. It is one of the best oils for treating sore and stiff muscles. As an antispasmodic agent, it is useful in easing cramping.

A strong antibacterial and antiviral agent, Sweet Marjoram oil helps to decongest the sinuses and fight off colds and flu. These properties also make it ideal for adding to the rinse water when cleaning off counters.

Sweet Marjoram oil is very effective in helping you relax. Mix three drops with two drops each of Chamomile and Lavender oils; it will help to ease headaches.

TEA TREE

Melaleuca alternifolia

Tea Tree oil has a very strong scent that may be overpowering. Still, it is an extremely useful oil to have on hand. This is the only oil, aside from Lavender, that can be applied directly to the skin.

This is another of the oils with exceptionally strong antibacterial, antifungal, and antiviral properties. Two drops each of Tea Tree and Eucalyptus oils used together make an exceptional treatment for colds and flu.

You can also use the oil to treat cuts and scrapes. If you have a fungal infection, such as ringworm or athlete's foot, you can apply Tea Tree oil directly to the spot a few times a day for effective relief.

Tea Tree oil is also great for disinfecting your home.

Home and First-Aid Recipes

ALL-PURPOSE DISINFECTANT

Use this delightful smelling mixture to clean and disinfect your kitchen naturally!

   15 drops Peppermint oil

   15 drops Eucalyptus oil

Mix this into your rinse water when wiping down your counters or cleaning the floors. If you have an ant problem, this is especially effective because ants cannot stand the smell of mint.

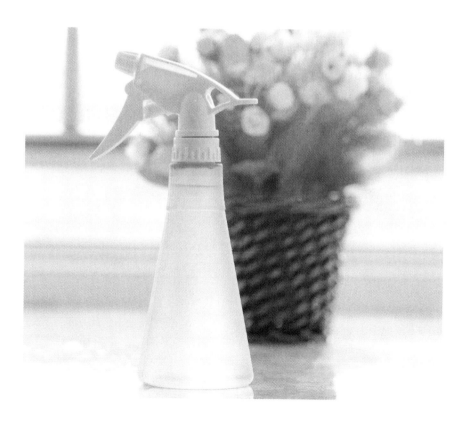

BATHE AWAY THE FLU

If you have high blood pressure or suffer from epilepsy, skip the Epsom salt and run a tepid bath. If you are pregnant, this exact treatment is not for you but can be used without the Eucalyptus and Tea Tree and with only one drop of sweet marjoram.

> 60 ml carrier oil
>
> 5 drops Eucalyptus essential oil
>
> 5 drops Tea Tree essential oil
>
> 5 drops Sweet Marjoram essential oil
>
> ½ cup baking soda
>
> 1 cup Epsom salt

Mix together the essential oils while drawing a bath. Rub about three-quarters of the mixture onto your body. Add baking soda and Epsom salt to the water, and stir to dissolve. The Epsom salt will relax any aching muscles. The water should be as hot as you can manage. Soak in the water for a minimum of 20 minutes. Keep a cool glass of plain water with you and drink it while you soak.

Dry yourself and rub the remaining essential oil blend onto your feet, chest, and throat. Wrap up very warmly before climbing into bed.

BUGS BE GONE

Keep away pests and smell delicious by using this natural bug repellent. Plus, you can avoid all of the harsh chemicals in conventional bug repellents.

    5 drops Citronella oil

    5 drops Basil oil

    400 ml water

    100 ml vodka

Mix all the ingredients well and spray as needed. Shake well before spraying each time.

CARPET FRESHENER

The baking soda in this recipe helps to soak up stale smells in the carpet and the essential oils lightly scent it.

    2 drops Lavender oil

    2 drops Chamomile oil

    1 cup baking soda

Mix together the oils and baking soda until completely combined. Sprinkle the mixture onto your carpets and allow it to stand for at least an hour or, better still, overnight.

DISINFECTING ROOM SPRITZ

Don't worry about the scent of the vodka in this recipe—it is pretty much odorless.

> 2 drops Lavender oil
>
> 2 drops Basil oil
>
> 2 drops Tea Tree oil
>
> 100 ml vodka (optional but fixes the scent)
>
> 400 ml water

Mix the ingredients well, place the spritz in an atomizer bottle, and spray as needed. Shake well before spraying each time.

LAUNDRY FRESHENER

Delight and soothe your senses with this intoxicating and simple way to freshen your linens and clothing.

> 250 ml plain water
>
> 15 drops Lavender oil

Mix together well in a spray bottle. If you hang out your laundry, spritz a light spray of the mixture when the laundry is almost dry. If you use a dryer, spritz the laundry just before putting it in.

As an alternative, you can add a few drops of Lavender oil to the rinse water in your washing machine.

PEACEFUL NIGHT CANDLE

If you want to benefit from aromatherapy but don't have a diffuser or an aromatherapy burner, a candle is a great place to start.

> 5 drops Lavender oil
>
> 5 drops Chamomile oil
>
> 1 large candle

Light your candle and allow it to burn until the wax begins to pool. Then add a few drops of the oils to the pooled wax. As the candle burns, the essential oil is heated and the scent is released. You will need to add more drops of the oils every now and then.

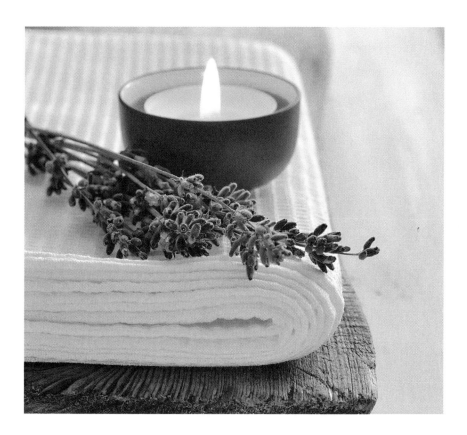

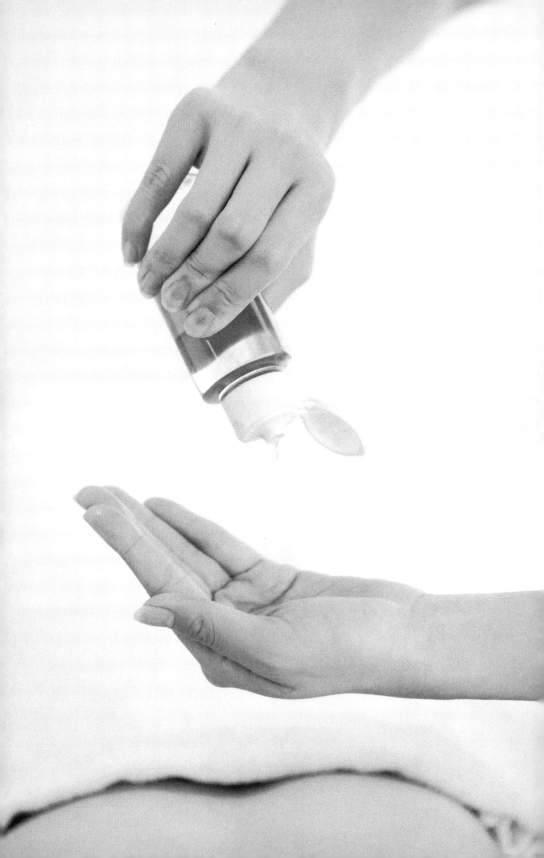

Chapter 8

Immune Health and Allergy Treatment with Essential Oils

"It has become evident that essential oils, both through topical application and inhalation, can positively impact the immune system by improving mood, increasing brain activity, and enhancing other biological functions important to health and healing."

—Jane Buckle, author of *Clinical Aromatherapy*

f you are as big a fan of essential oils as I am, I hope you discover new oils to add to your medicine cabinet for a refreshing change from your usual treatments. Just pick one or two, as many overlap in their benefits.

MASSAGE is considered to be an effective method to strengthen the immune system, as it combines essential oil application with touch, entering through the largest organ in our bodies, our skin:

* For a full-body massage, put 12 drops of essential oil in 2 ounces of carrier oil or fragrance-free, natural lotion.

* For a neck and shoulder massage, put 12 drops of essential oil in 1 ounce of carrier oil or fragrance-free, natural lotion.

* For a foot massage, put 10–25 drops of essential oil in 1 ounce of carrier oil or fragrance-free, natural lotion. Massage your feet and cover them with cotton socks before going to sleep.

* Other places to apply essential oils include the back of the neck/skull base, pulse points, and behind the ears.

Essential Oils for Allergies

FOUR SINGLE-NOTE OILS FOR ALLERGIES

* Basil essential oil helps reduce inflammation and fight infections for people who frequently suffer from allergic reactions. It contains eugenol compounds that are effective in eliminating various bacterial and fungal infections. This can help to prevent yeast or mold from infecting your respiratory tract, triggering asthma attacks. It's very helpful for the treatment of asthma and related conditions. Studies have shown that basil also acts as an antihistamine in reducing the body's allergic response. It's traditionally used to alleviate coughs, headaches, and gastrointestinal upset. It also has a calming effect and helps you sleep better.

* Roman Chamomile essential oil is a great remedy for a wide range of allergic reactions and a number of inflammatory conditions. It's the perfect essential oil to relieve allergic skin reactions. Asthma or hay fever sufferers often have outbreaks of hives with dry, red, itchy patches of skin. Chamomile is wonderful as a topical application (combined with a carrier oil or a fragrance-free, natural lotion) for fast relief from dermatitis. Inhaling Chamomile essential oil in a diffuser can also have a calming effect on your respiratory system when you're suffering from sneezing, blocked sinuses, or excess mucus. It can also help relieve sinus headaches and treat bacterial infections. And for an allergic food reaction with an upset stomach, abdominal pain, nausea, and/or vomiting, a cup of chamomile tea will soothe your discomfort.

* Rosemary essential oil is slightly milder than Eucalyptus oil, but it also works to alleviate inflammation in the sinuses. A 2011 study found that

Rosemary essential oil also has antimicrobial properties and can neutralize some pathogens. It's an expectorant that is good for fighting colds, sinusitis, rhinitis, and bronchitis, and expands and deepens breathing.

* Sandalwood essential oil can help relieve your symptoms if you suffer from pet allergies, dust allergies, or allergic rhinitis. It helps reduce the effect of allergens and the reaction of antibodies in your system. Breathing in sandalwood vapors helps counter runny noses, stuffiness, and mucus.

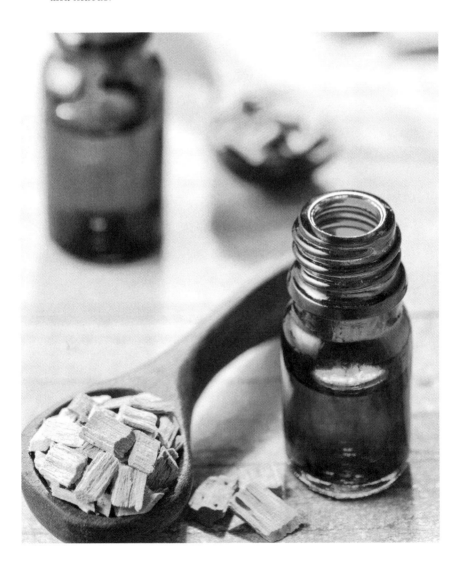

Three Combination Oil Blends for Allergies

Combination oils may be blended with a carrier oil or a fragrance-free natural lotion and the whole mix put in a roll-on bottle. Alternatively, you can place a few drops in a diffuser.

* Almond, Geranium, and Sandalwood essential oils: Massaging with three drops each of these oils for five minutes daily for seven days yields significant improvements in allergy symptoms.

* Frankincense, Sandalwood, and Ravensara essential oils: This combination is good for people suffering from perennial allergic rhinitis. It helps open up nasal passages, and also clears up runny, itchy noses and sneezing. Use two drops of each in Almond oil as the carrier. Mix and diffuse into the air. Ravensara essential oil has health benefits as an analgesic, anti-allergenic, antibacterial, antimicrobial, antidepressant, antifungal, antiseptic, antispasmodic, antiviral, aphrodisiac, disinfectant, diuretic, expectorant, relaxant, and tonic substance. Frankincense essential oil is an expectorant, and an antimicrobial and antitussive (that is, it relieves coughing).

* Lemon, Lavender, and Peppermint essential oils: Measure equal amounts of Lavender and Lemon essential oils and then add half the amount of Peppermint and diffuse or mix with a carrier oil of your choice and rub on feet.

Three Healing Recipes for Allergies

LEMONGRASS ALLERGY RELIEF

Makes ¼ cup

This recipe will stimulate your system to optimally respond to allergens. The Lemongrass will tonify your immune system to produce less histamine and therefore lessen allergy symptoms. The Clove oil is warming and stimulating and will alleviate many allergy symptoms. It is also mildly antibacterial and therefore prevents other immune upset.

> 10–15 drops Lemon Grass oil
>
> 3 drops Clove oil
>
> ¼ cup (or desired quantity) Sweet Almond oil

Place the Lemongrass oil and the Clove oil in a 10 ml roll-on bottle, then fill it to the top with Sweet Almond oil. Shake it well before use and roll it on your chest and cheeks. Keep it away from your eyes and nasal openings.

To diffuse, put 5 or 6 drops in the diffuser for a fresh, invigorating scent. To use it as a sleep aid, put a drop on your pillow at night or on the palms of your hands. Yields about ¼ cup. Any leftover mixture can be massaged into feet and legs.

LEMON-PEPPERMINT MIST

Makes 20 to 30 treatments

This blend of essential oils eases inflammation and strengthens the immune system, making allergies less troublesome. It can be used several times a day, and has a fresh, delicious fragrance.

Lavender oil

Lemon oil

Peppermint oil

4 ounces purified water

30 drops Lavender oil

30 drops Lemon oil

30 drops Peppermint oil

Put in a dark-colored glass spray bottle. Shake well to blend. Spray this blend throughout any indoor spaces where allergy sufferers spend time. Repeat as many times as needed. Shake the bottle before each use.

NASAL ALLERGY IRRIGATION

Makes 1 treatment

This is a simple, effective treatment that helps reduce the inflammation that accompanies severe allergies.

  8 ounces warm purified water

  ¼ teaspoon fine salt

  5 drops Lavender essential oil

  5 drops Lemon essential oil

  3 drops Peppermint essential oil

In a neti pot, place the water and salt.

Add to that the Lavender, Lemon, and Peppermint essential oils.

Stir to blend all the ingredients. Using the neti pot, perform nasal irrigation, then gently blow your nose. You can repeat this treatment up to three times a day to relieve allergy symptoms considerably. Don't use this with children under 12 years old unless they can tolerate a neti pot. Be sure to sanitize your neti pot before each use.

Essential Oils for Your Immune System

Five Single-Note Oils to Boost Your Immune System

* Bay Laurel essential oil boosts the immune system, protecting you from infections. It's a tonic, an antiseptic, an antibiotic, an antineuralgic, an antispasmodic, an analgesic, an astringent, an emmenagogue, a febrifuge, an insecticide, a sedative, a stomachic, and a sudorific. Its many properties are beneficial for the whole body. It strengthens the liver, stomach, and the intestines, while improving the metabolic functions, such as the breakdown of food and the absorption of nutrients. It promotes proper excretion, regulates the endocrine system's hormones and modulates enzymes. It also provides emotional benefits, as it bolsters the nervous system, and alleviates fever, infection, and pain.

* Frankincense essential oil can boost the immune system and fight off bladder cancer. Two studies from 2009 and 2014 found that frankincense appears to distinguish cancerous cells from normal bladder cells and that it kills off bladder cancer cells. It also has anti-inflammatory properties, which may be useful in the treatment of autoimmune disorders, along with antiseptic, expectorant, and decongestant properties that boost the immune system. In India, frankincense has long been used as a rejuvenating medicine because it helps clear the lungs and other mucus-related problems. It's helpful in relieving stress, too: It has been shown to reduce heart rate and high blood pressure.

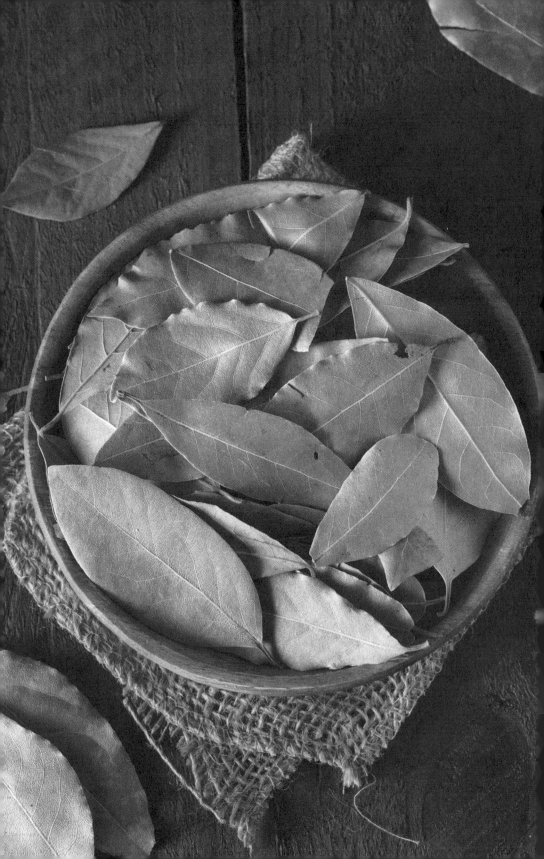

* Niaouli essential oil boosts the immune system because of its expectorant and decongestant properties. It may be used to treat the common cold, whooping cough, the flu, bronchitis, sinusitis, catarrh, asthma, pneumonia, laryngitis, coughing, sore throat, tuberculosis, and other respiratory infections. It helps clear congestion and open up blocked nasal passages that are saturated with phlegm and mucous. Niaouli essential oil may also be able to bring down a fever by treating infections inside the body and promoting sweat. Adding a few drops with a carrier oil to your bath can help fight off intestinal parasites, such as tapeworms and roundworms.

* Parsley essential oil has vitamins, minerals, and antioxidants that help strengthen the immune system, such as vitamin C, vitamin A, vitamin K, folate, and niacin. Vitamin A acts directly on white blood cells. The chlorophyll in parsley has antibacterial and antifungal properties. And studies have shown that parsley contains antioxidant and antibacterial properties as well.

* Thyme essential oil supports the immune, respiratory, digestive, nervous, and other bodily systems. It is one of the most ancient medicinal herbs on record and one of the strongest antioxidants known. It has large amounts of thymol, which give it its antiseptic, antibacterial, antispasmodic, and hypertensive properties. It's wonderful for women experiencing menstrual and menopause symptoms, as it balances hormone levels. It keeps the body protected from dangerous diseases and conditions, such as stroke, arthritis, fungal and bacterial infections, and skin irritations.

Three Combination Oil Ideas for Your Immune System

Combination oils may be blended with a carrier oil or a fragrance-free, natural lotion, and the whole mix put in a roll-on bottle, or a few drops may be placed in a diffuser.

* Bay Laurel, Frankincense, and Thyme oils in equal amounts.

* Sage, Black Pepper, and Manuka oils in equal amounts.

* Niaouli and Peppermint oils: 3 drops Niaouli oil to 1 drop Peppermint oil.

Recipes to Boost Your Immune System

ANTIBACTERIAL AND ANTIVIRAL DIFFUSION BLEND

Yields 1 capsule

This combination is renowned for its ability to keep sickness at bay. At the very least, this diffusion is likely to lessen symptoms and shorten their duration.

Lavender essential oil

Tea Tree essential oil

Thyme essential oil

In a dark-colored glass bottle, large enough to hold the amount of the diffusion blend you want to make, combine equal amounts of Lavender, Tea Tree, and Thyme essential oils, and shake well to blend. Store the bottle in a cool, dark place between uses.

ANTIBIOTIC REPLACEMENT RECIPE

Yields 1 treatment

This is the exact recipe I use in any situation where a doctor would prescribe an antibiotic or when I feel as if I am fighting off a serious infection. I also use this if I think I might have been exposed to pathogens or germs. If someone around me has been sick, or if I traveled on a plane and people were sneezing and coughing during flu season, I immediately take this remedy. I have used this formula myself to treat fungal infections, colds, and eye and ear infections over the years.

When taking this blend internally, make sure you are using the highest-quality therapeutic grade oils. It's important to completely encapsulate this blend in a vegetable capsule before swallowing. If you try to drink this in liquid form in any kind of carrier—be it water, juice, or almond milk—it is likely to irritate your stomach. It needs to be in a capsule with no oil on the outside of the capsule before being swallowed. This is potent stuff!

2¾ parts Thyme oil

2 parts Oregano oil

1½ parts Sage oil

1 part Lemon Balm oil

Fill one capsule with the prescribed parts of each oil.

AROMATHERAPY STEAM TO CLEAR THE UPPER RESPIRATORY TRACT

Yields 1 treatment

Get ready to get steamy! Invite good health by treating your sinuses to an invigorating and expansive steam with these healing scents.

Boil 2 cups of water, pour into a ceramic bowl, and add:

1 drop Tea Tree oil

1 drop Eucalyptus oil

1 drop Peppermint oil

Cover your head with a towel, lean over the bowl, and breathe deeply for 5 minutes. If it hurts, you know the oils are attacking infected cells. And to top it off, you now you look like your great-grandmother with her head in a towel!

BLACK PEPPER AND BERGAMOT BATH

Black pepper is an excellent overall tonic for good spleen and colon function. Its antiseptic properties keep colds, the flu, and the blues away. Bergamot has the same effect and also lifts the spirits.

> 1 tablespoon carrier oil or fragrance-free, natural lotion
>
> 6 drops Black Pepper essential oil
>
> 6 drops Bergamot essential oil

In a small glass bowl, pour the carrier oil, along with the Black Pepper and Bergamot essential oils, and stir to combine. As you are running the bathwater, pour in the entire mixture and soak in this lovely fragrant bath for at least 15 minutes.

IMMUNE-BOOSTING FOOT MASSAGE

Yields just over a ¼ cup

This mixture can effectively treat colds and infections if used three times per day for five to seven days. It smells delightful and enters your body effectively through the skin on your feet.

> ¼ cup Coconut oil
>
> 10 drops Oregano essential oil
>
> 2 drops each of Orange, Clove, Cinnamon Bark/Leaf, Eucalyptus, and Rosemary oils

Place the Coconut oil and the essential oils in a roll-on bottle.

Close it and apply as needed to the soles of your feet.

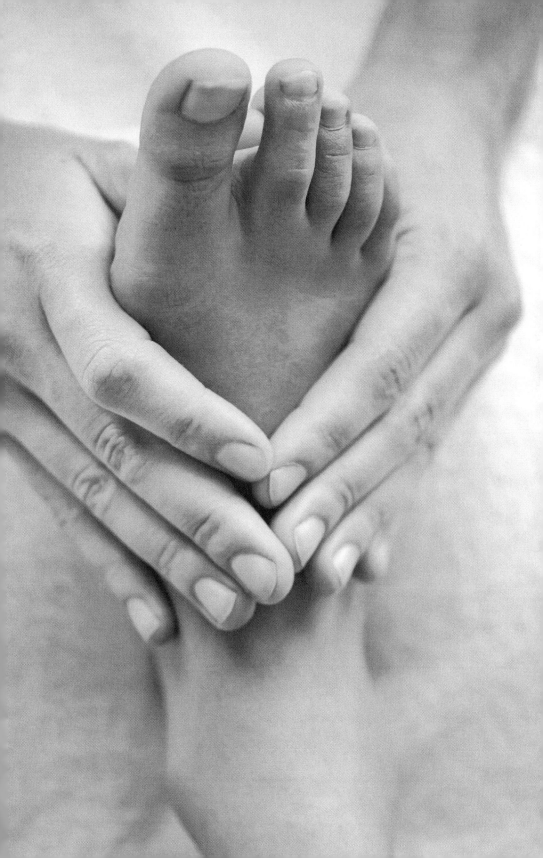

OIL-PULLING IMMUNE-HEALTH MOUTHWASH

Yields 1 ounce

So much of our health begins in our mouth! It is where we take in our food and begin the digestive process through chewing and the breaking down of food through saliva secretions. The health of our gums and teeth is directly connected to our heart health and our immune health. The process of oil pulling has been around for thousands of years and has been used in Indian culture for a long time. It is now recommended by many dentists. Oil pulling is believed to help remove bacteria, fungi, and even viruses from the gum line. It's also believed to pull heavy metals from the body in a safe way and encapsulate them in the Coconut oil that you will spit out when you're done.

Organic, high-quality Coconut oil

Cinnamon Bark oil

Clove oil

Lemon oil

Cinnamon leaf oil

Rosemary oil

Eucalyptus oil

Use a jar to store your mouthwash. You can prepare it in the same jar. If you'd like to make a sizable quantity, you can use a 14-ounce jar of Coconut oil. Remove a couple teaspoons of the oil to make room for your additional ingredients. Run the jar under warm water until the Coconut oil liquefies. One of the great things about Coconut oil is it becomes more solid at a lower temperature—right around 76°F.

Once you liquefy the oil add 5 drops of the Cinnamon Bark, Clove, Lemon, and Cinnamon Leaf oils. Add 3 drops of Rosemary oil and 2 drops of Eucalyptus oil. Stir the mixture thoroughly then place it in the refrigerator. Once it resolidifies, you most likely will not have to store it in the fridge. As long as your bathroom is 76°F or cooler, you can keep it right there. I recommend using a clean spoon to remove about a teaspoon of the mixture after brushing your teeth. Allow the solid to melt in your mouth and then swish the oil blend around thoroughly in all areas of your mouth for 10–20 minutes.

When you are finished, make sure to spit the oil in the trash and not down the drain because it may clog. Oil pulling is recommended to be done on an empty stomach. Do not do it right after you eat because it may cause nausea. It's very pleasant and many people find it relaxing before bedtime.

TEA TREE OIL VAGINAL SUPPOSITORY

Yield depends on the size of mold

This remedy is one of the most effective ways to treat vaginal yeast and bacterial infections. It can be used for bacterial vaginosis (also known as BV) and to treat Candida infections of the reproductive tract. Additionally, if you are treating fungal and bacterial infections in other parts of the body and you want to safeguard your reproductive system, you can use this treatment as a preventative, especially if you are already prone to yeast or bacterial infections in this area.

> Organic high-quality coconut oil
> Organic therapeutic grade tea tree oil

You will need something to use as a mold for your suppositories. You can use an ice cube tray with small ice cube openings. You will only fill the openings about halfway and will be placing your mold filled with ingredients in the freezer after preparation, so clear a spot and make sure to have some plastic wrap or parchment paper on hand to cover the molds because you don't want any debris falling in there.

Use about 2 teaspoons of coconut oil and run the jar under warm water to liquefy the oil. Place the liquefied oil in each opening in the mold and then add to 2–6 drops of Tea Tree oil per suppository. Using a toothpick or stir, stick-mix the two oils. Cover and place in the freezer overnight.

To use, remove one suppository and use in the evening. Put on a pair of cotton underwear after insertion to catch the oil as it melts out throughout the night. You may want to line your mold or ice cube tray with plastic wrap so you can more easily remove the suppositories.

When you insert a suppository, try to put it in quickly so it doesn't melt outside the body. Ideally, you want to insert in, then lay down so it can melt on the inside and stay in there for a while before it drips out.

This remedy can also be useful for women who frequently exercise and sweat a lot. Sometimes this can throw off vaginal flora and promote bacterial vaginosis. But, you can insert a tea tree suppository before your workout. Just make sure to wear cotton underwear under your workout gear to catch the oil.

The company Tea Tree Therapy Inc. makes an excellent suppository with Tea Tree oil for vaginal hygiene if you would like to purchase this recipe pre-made.

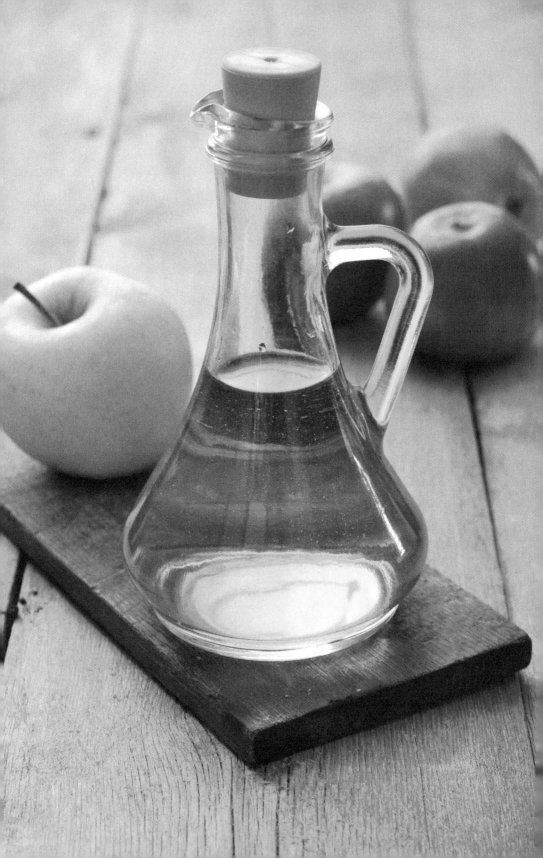

Quick and Easy Immune-Boosting, Anti-Allergy Drinks

ACV CITRUS DELIGHT

Yields 2 ounces

This is a great natural remedy that wards off all types of allergies. The trick is to use it on a consistent basis. It keeps your body alkaline, maintains your pH balance, and strengthens your immunity.

MIX:

> 1 tablespoon apple cider vinegar
>
> 1 tablespoon freshly squeezed lemon juice
>
> 2 drops Orange Peel essential oil
>
> ½ tablespoon raw honey

Drink this three times a day.

INVIGORATING ORANGE-LEMON GREEN TEA

Drink a cup whole leaf green tea with a drop of Orange essential oil and a drop of Lemon essential oil hot or cold. This tea has an antioxidant (EGCG) that blocks the production of histamine and immunoglobulin E, both of which trigger allergy symptoms. The more green tea you drink, the more the allergic reactions are suppressed. Green tea has an anti-inflammatory effect on the immune system.

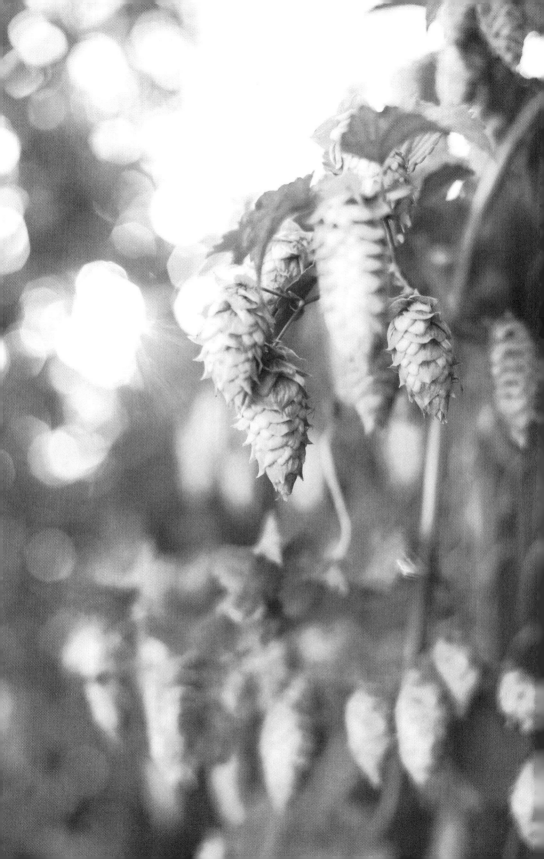

Chapter 9

Neurological and Emotional Health and Essential Oils

When it comes to neurological and emotional health, research has proven what traditional wisdom held to be true all along: essential oils have a profound healing effect. We still don't fully understand why essential oils have such an impact on the mind and the emotions, but it is clear that they do.

What we do know is that there are two olfactory nerve centers that connect with the limbic system. The limbic system is the part of the brain that controls emotion and memory. This connection is the reason that just a whiff of a familiar smell can evoke a strong emotional response and/or bring memories flooding back.

According to research conducted in England and Japan, we have two different responses to odors—hardwired responses and soft-wired responses. Hardwired responses are entirely instinctual. By contrast, soft-wired responses are based on your life experience. So, for example, the scent of the perfume your mother used to wear all the time would evoke a soft-wired response.

So when it comes to essential oils, are the responses hard- or soft-wired? Will the oils work in the same manner for everyone who uses them? That is, will they all have the same effect?

Emotional responses to a particular scent are soft-wired, so your personal response is going to depend a great deal on your own experiences and circumstances. While we know that oils have certain general properties, the effect on each individual may differ.

Interestingly, the pharmacological responses will be very similar from one person to the next, but the psychological effects may differ substantially. You psychological response may depend on the method of application, the concentration of the essential oil, the circumstances under which the essential oil is used, whether or not you like the smell, and whether or not you are able to smell certain scents.

This is why it's important to use essential oils whose scent you enjoy. From a psychological perspective, whether or not you like the smell will be more important than the inherent healing properties of the essential oil.

TRY BEFORE YOU BUY

To ensure that you like the scent of a particular oil, you should sniff a tester beforehand. The more you like the scent, the more likely you are to use the oil and the more likely it is to have a positive effect on your psyche.

When you have a selection of oils that you like, you can start blending them and creating even more potent remedies. Once you get the blends right, the oils in the blend will enhance each other, heightening the healing properties of the blend.

To create harmonious blends, mix together scents that belong to the same basic classification or family. For example, Sweet Orange and Bergamot oils go together well because they are both citrus oils.

There are some classic blends that also work well together, such as citrus and spice oils or citrus and wood oils. So Sweet Orange also works well with Sandalwood oil or Black Pepper oil.

HOW BEST TO USE OILS FOR THE MIND

How you use oils to lift your mood and calm your mind will depend on what your particular circumstance is. Diffusing the oils is a quick and easy way to enjoy their benefits. You would normally require around about half an hour's exposure to the oils to feel the full effect when diffusing them.

If your muscles are very tense, it is useful to use the oils in the bath or as a body rub. When using them in the bath, draw the bath and mix the oils first with a teaspoon of organic milk. Pour this into the bathwater just before you climb into it. (The fat in the milk will help to disperse the oils.) Don't use more than five or six drops of oil in your bath or you could risk irritating your skin.

If you're applying the oils topically, you should first mix them into a carrier oil, such as Grape Seed oil or Sweet Almond oil, or an organic aqueous base. The oils should make up no more than 3 percent of the overall mixture.

Another way to use the oils is to apply them in a cold compress. To do this, take a bowl of cool water, add two or three drops of the oil, and soak a clean washcloth in the water. Wring the water out and apply it as necessary. If you are trying to get rid of a headache, applying one compress on the forehead and another on the back of the neck is helpful.

If you want to use the oils discreetly at work, place a tissue into a sealable container. Place a few drops of the oils that you want to use onto the tissue and seal the container. Carry it with you and take a sniff when necessary.

OILS FOR THE MIND

There are many different oils that have a beneficial effect on your mind. You can choose oils that are best related to your particular condition.

BERGAMOT
Citrus bergamia

Bergamot helps to keep you grounded and to balance the emotions. It is gently uplifting and can help to treat depression.

FRANKINCENSE
Boswellia carteri

Frankincense has a long tradition of use for inducing a meditative state. It helps to reduce anxiety and tension, and is also very uplifting. If you are feeling restless or overwhelmed, Frankincense is a great oil to use. Concentrated boswellia is taken for pain relief and prevention, specifically for nerve pain. The oil can be used for pain relief as well.

GERANIUM
Pelargonium graveolens

Geranium is calming and uplifting at the same time. This makes it extremely useful in warding off depression and tension caused by stress.

During times of grief, this is one of the most helpful oils.

It is useful in promoting deep relaxation and can assist in clearing up your complexion, especially when outbreaks are related to stress.

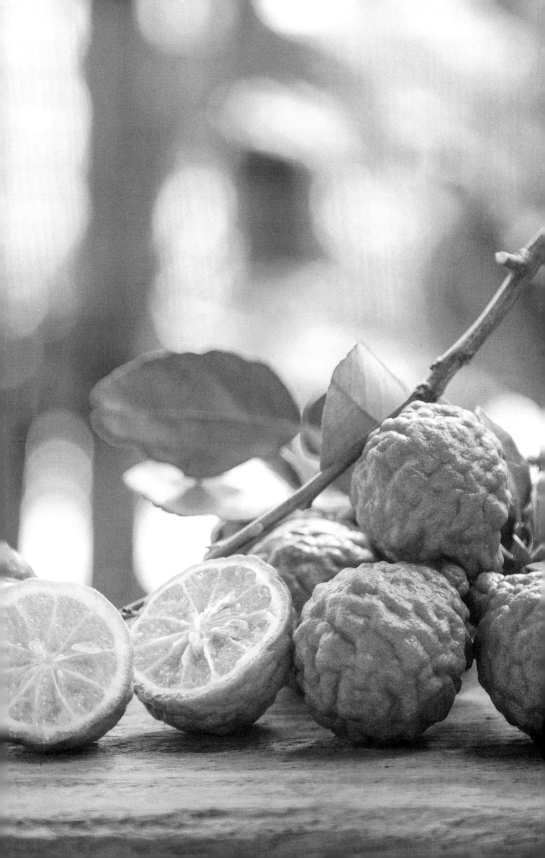

GERMAN CHAMOMILE

Matricaria recutita

Chamomile oil helps to calm nervous tension and promote deep relaxation. Blend three drops with one drop of Lavender oil, or even on its own, it is an excellent oil when you are struggling to relax or to fall asleep.

If you suffer from tension headaches, a cold compress with chamomile will alleviate your pain.

If you have very tight muscles as a result of tension, Chamomile oil can be applied, diluted in a carrier oil, to help with pain relief.

Chamomile has strong analgesic and sedative properties. You can boost its overall effectiveness by blending it with equal parts Lavender oil. A few drops of each will work wonders.

HOPS

Humulus lupulus

Hops are useful for more than just making beer. The oil acts as a sedative, so it's very effective at helping you relax. It will ease nervous tension and headaches, and can counter insomnia.

Neuralgia responds well to the topical application of hops, as long as it is diluted.

JASMINE

Jasminum officinale

Jasmine is one of the best oils to use if you are feeling apathetic or depressed. It induces a sense of euphoria and can help to restore optimism and a lust for life. It also builds healthful energy in your kidneys, which results in increased sexual potency and promotes aphrodisiac qualities.

LAVENDER

Lavandula angustifolia

Lavender is an all-around nerve tonic. It will help you to relax when you are feeling stressed and will help you to nod off faster and enjoy a more restful night's sleep.

Lavender oil is excellent in treating shock and is uplifting for those suffering from depression.

It is highly useful as a cure for headaches, especially those caused by nervous tension. You can rub a drop of the oil into each temple at the onset of a migraine to stop it in its tracks.

It partners very well with equal parts of Chamomile oil to create a deeply relaxing blend.

Lavender does have quite a strong scent, so be sure to try it before you buy it.

LEMON BALM

Melissa officinalis

This is a great oil for treating depression and anxiety. Be sure to look for a reputable blend, though, because it is often adulterated with Lemongrass and Lemongrass has very different properties.

Lemon Balm will help soothe tension and anxiety. It is useful in treating headaches and migraines and makes a good remedy for shock as well.

MARJORAM, SWEET

Origanum majorana

Marjoram is exceptional at easing tense muscles. It has deeply relaxing properties and can ward off insomnia, nervous tension, and headaches.

Blend two drops with an equal quantity of Vetiver oil; it makes an excellent muscle rub or addition to the bath.

NEROLI

Citrus aurantium var. amara

Neroli should be in your first aid kit. It is referred to as the "rescue remedy" of essential oils. Neroli is especially helpful when you are in shock or struggling to accept a loss.

Uplifting and helpful in easing depression and anxiety, Neroli is a balancing oil that works well if you suffer from mood swings.

ROSEMARY

Rosmarinus officinalis

If you are battling nervous exhaustion or debility related to stress, rosemary should be on your shopping list. You can also use it fight colds and infections.

It blends well with Lavender oil to make a potent headache cure, and has analgesic properties when applied topically. The more rosemary oil you use the more potent your blend will be, so you can vary the quantity by how strong you want the healing properties to be. For example, if you use two drops each of rosemary and lavender, then you will create an effective and moderate blend. If you choose to use four drops of rosemary and two of lavender, then you will create a stronger blend with greater beneficial properties for the nervous and immune systems. If you do not want to overwhelm yourself and are feeling sensitive, then you might choose two forms of rosemary and four of lavender.

Rosemary can cause uterine contractions, so it is best avoided during pregnancy.

SWEET ORANGE

Citrus sinensis

Sweet Orange oil has a fresh scent that boosts your spirits. It also helps to build up your energy levels.

VALERIAN

Valeriana fauriei

Valerian is an herb that has been used for a long time as a general sedative and relaxant. The essential oil eases insomnia, headaches, and nervous indigestion brought on by stress. It is also a good oil to use if you are struggling with restlessness.

VETIVER

Vetiveria zizanioides

If stress is making it difficult for you to do anything, vetiver will help you regain control. It is extremely relaxing and has a deep, earthy aroma. It is especially good for easing tense muscles and can help you overcome depression.

YLANG-YLANG

Cananga odorata var. genuina

Ylang-ylang has long been noted for its aphrodisiac properties, but it is also an oil that induces a state of deep relaxation. It has uplifting qualities, making it useful in the treatment of depression, and it also counteracts insomnia.

It should be noted that it has a very pervasive scent, and this can be overpowering if used excessively.

Oils Blends for Your Mind and Heart

ANTISTRESS DIFFUSION

Yield: 1 treatment

    5 drops Neroli essential oil

    3 drops Petitgrain essential oil

    2 drops Bergamot essential oil

Mix everything together and diffuse.

BEDTIME DIFFUSION

Yield: 1 full diffuser

Scent your bedroom with this lush and relaxing blend of oils to promote relaxation and an open heart.

    6 drops Ylang-ylang essential oil

    6 drops Rose essential oil

    2 drops Vetiver essential oil

    1 drop Roman Chamomile essential oil

Mix everything together and diffuse.

CALM-ME-QUICK DIFFUSION

Yield: 1 treatment

Banish stress with this light and uplifting blend. Use throughout any day or stressful situation to calm your mind and promote feelings of well-being.

    6 drops Lavender essential oil

    4 drops Sweet Orange essential oil

    4 drops Bergamot essential oil

Mix everything together and diffuse.

COMPLETE DESTRESSING BLEND

Yield: 1 treatment

Use this blend to ease muscle tension from stress and overexertion. The clary sage included promotes clarity of mind, while the frankincense and germanium will help the nervous system balance itself with ease.

    2 tablespoons Sweet Almond oil

    5 drops Clary Sage essential oil

    5 drops Frankincense essential oil

    5 drops Geranium essential oil

Mix everything together and apply to tense muscles.

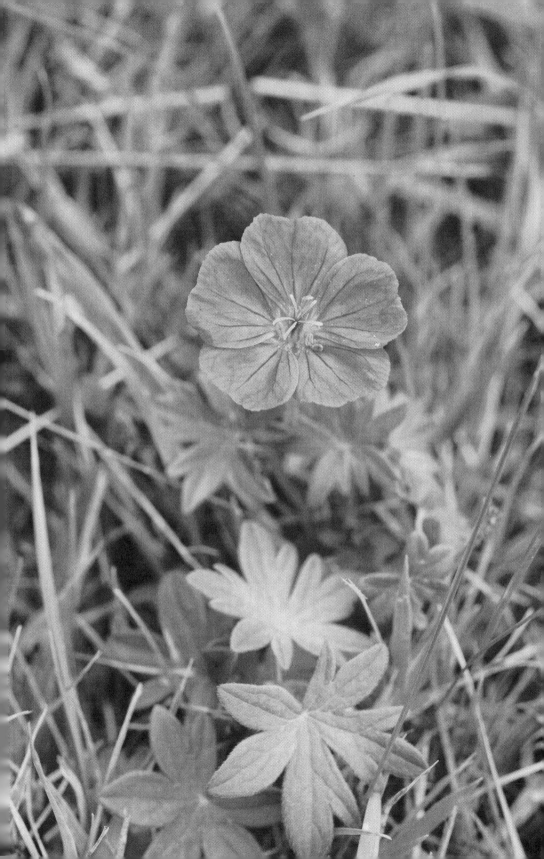

DEEP RELAXATION BLEND

Yield: 1 treatment

This blend will relax your heart and allow you to let go of old emotional wounds with ease. Use before sleep to heal your heart gently. As you fall asleep, say to yourself, "I relax my heart and shoulders and rest in emotional safety."

    2 tablespoons Sweet Almond oil

    4 drops Frankincense essential oil

    3 drops Rose absolute or essential oil

    1 drop Geranium essential oil

Mix everything together and apply to tense muscles.

DEPRESSION-BUSTING BATH

Yield: 1 treatment

This bath is grounding for the senses while also allowing your kidneys to detox in the hot water. The jasmine will promote healthy sexuality and the grapefruit will raise your spirits.

    1 tablespoon Sweet Almond oil or whole milk

    2 drops Sandalwood essential oil

    2 drops Jasmine absolute or essential oil

    1 drop Grapefruit essential oil

Mix everything together and add to your bathwater.

ME-TIME MIX

Yield: 1 treatment

Treat yourself to this exotic room enhancing blend. It is the perfect accompaniment to creative endeavors and will ignite your imagination.

    5 drops Frankincense essential oil

    3 drops Neroli essential oil

    2 drops Mandarin essential oil

Mix everything together and diffuse.

SUNSHINE DIFFUSION

Yield: 1 treatment

Wake up your senses with this bright and cheerful blend. Fill your space with enthusiasm and positivity using this mix in your diffuser.

    5 drops Lemon Balm essential oil

    3 drops Lemon essential oil

    3 drops Cypress essential oil

    2 drops Bergamot essential oil

Mix everything together and diffuse.

You can bolster your neurological and emotional health using essential oils, without all the negative side effects that you get from medication. Use nature's gift to start living a happier, healthier life today.

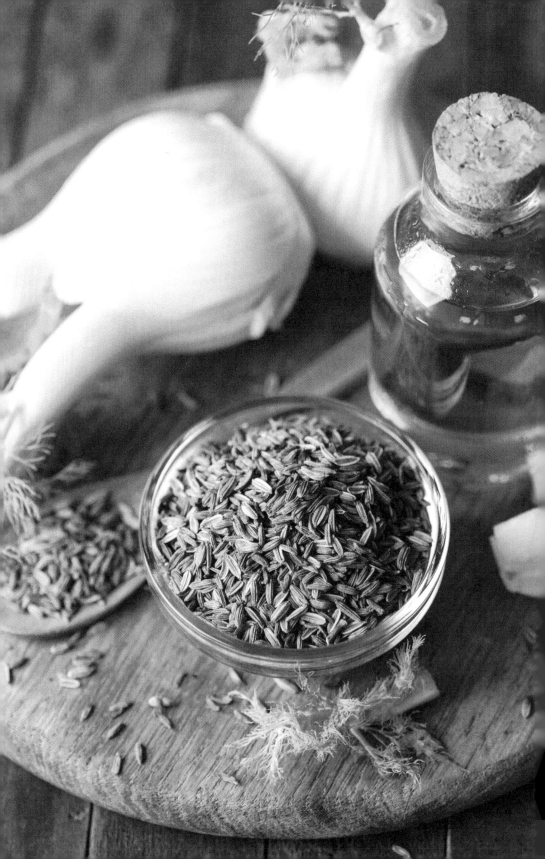

Chapter 10

Digestive and Endocrine System Healing with Essential Oils

"The therapeutic potential of essential oils, like other plant-derived remedies, has yet to be fully realized."

—Julia Lawless, author of the *Encyclopedia of Essential Oils*

Essential oils are popular aromatics for scenting a space or setting a mood, but they can be so much more beneficial to our health. We are just at the tip of the iceberg in terms of learning how essential oils can affect our bodies.

Modern science is recognizing that essential oils can have a beneficial effect on multiple systems in the body. While you should consult a doctor for all your medical needs, certain common ailments can be soothed with the use of essential oils in the home. This chapter focuses on treating common issues with the digestive, reproductive and endocrine systems in your body, such as indigestion, menstrual cramps, and other everyday ailments.

THE DIGESTIVE SYSTEM

Digestion is common to all of us. This bodily system consists of the esophagus, the stomach, and the small and large intestines. It also includes organs that aid in digestion: the tongue, the salivary glands, the pancreas, and the liver. It's a familiar process all of us engage in every day. You eat food, the food gets digested to extract nutrients, and then you excrete the waste. You're probably digesting right now!

You're also probably pretty familiar with the downsides of having a digestive system. Consuming greasy, sugary junk food, an excess amount of food, or even just food that disagrees with your body can lead to gas, nausea, bloating, and cramping. You might suffer pain and discomfort for an evening or even days at a time. Essential oils can alleviate these everyday ailments. The following essential oils can be helpful in supporting your recovery from digestion woes:

BASIL: Relaxes muscles; improves digestion; alleviates constipation and bloating, plus pain from indigestion and nausea

BLACK PEPPER: Eases constipation, diarrhea, gas

CARDAMOM: Supports healthy digestion and a healthy stomach

CHAMOMILE: Relaxes muscles; alleviates pain from indigestion, diarrhea, and gas

CORIANDER: Alleviates nausea, vomiting, and diarrhea

FENNEL: Reduces the pain of indigestion; alleviates gas, constipation, and diarrhea

GINGER: Treats stomachache, nausea, pain from indigestion, diarrhea

LEMONGRASS: Relieves muscle pain, reduces stomachache, alleviates gas and digestion, reduces inflammation

PEPPERMINT: Provides muscle pain relief; alleviates bloating, gas, and nausea, plus pain from indigestion

These essential oils can best support your digestive system when diluted in an oil to be applied externally or when diffused for aromatherapy purposes. Use the recipes below to set yourself on the path to happier digestion.

Blends for Happier Digestion

BLOATING RELIEF BLEND

Bloating can turn a fun evening out with friends or a productive afternoon at work into a painful and uncomfortable ordeal. A discreet application of this Bloating Relief Blend can help get you back to enjoying your free time or crunching those numbers at work. This blend of essential oils should help reduce your bloating and ease your pain and discomfort. Try sipping some peppermint tea if you have some on hand to help further ease the bloating.

> Fennel essential oil
> Peppermint essential oil
> Basil essential oil
> Carrier oil

Mix 2 drops of Fennel essential oil with 1 drop each of Peppermint and Basil essential oils and a tablespoon of your favorite carrier oil such as Jojoba, Coconut, or Almond oil to dilute. When the ingredients are combined, dab some on your finger and rub into your stomach, abdomen, or the soles of your feet. You can store this blend in a dark-colored, airtight jar, and keep it at your desk at work for discreet relief.

INDIGESTION PAIN BLEND

A bout of indigestion is the worst. The discomfort and pain from intestines in distress can leave you feeling awkward and out of sorts, especially if you're in a situation where you can't leave right away. This Indigestion Pain Blend can be rubbed on your stomach, abdomen, or the soles of your feet to provide some relief.

Chamomile essential oil

Fennel essential oil

Basil essential oil

Ginger essential oil

Black Pepper essential oil

Carrier oil

Combine 2 drops each of Chamomile, Fennel, Basil, Ginger, and Black Pepper essential oils with a tablespoon of your favorite carrier oil. You can use Jojoba, Sweet Almond, Coconut, or any other oil that works well for you, as long as the essential oils get diluted. When the ingredients are combined, dab some of the blend on your finger and rub it onto your stomach, abdomen, or the soles of your feet. You can store this in a dark-colored, airtight jar and keep it at your desk at work for discreet relief. Pair this balm with a cup of your favorite ginger or peppermint tea to send more relief to your digestion system.

NAUSEA RELIEF BLEND

Ease your discomfort and soothe your roiling stomach in an easy way by breathing this Nausea Relief Blend of essential oils from your diffuser. The mix of essential oils should ease your upset stomach and provide some relief from whatever is ailing you. If you feel up to it, try sipping a mix of chamomile and peppermint or ginger tea to calm your stomach and get back on your feet.

Peppermint essential oil

Chamomile essential oil

Coriander essential oil

Cardamom essential oil

Ginger essential oil

Add the appropriate amount of water for your diffuser and 2 drops each of Peppermint, Chamomile, Coriander, Cardamom, and Ginger essential oils. Diffuse the oils into the air and inhale the healing, calming aroma.

Endocrine System

The endocrine system comprises a collection of glands that secrete hormones. These glands include the pineal gland, the hypothalamus, the thyroid gland, the parathyroid gland, the pituitary gland, the pancreas, the adrenal glands, and the ovaries/testicles. This system of glands works by secreting hormones into the circulatory system so they can travel directly to organs in the body. This process is known as "endocrine signaling."

You're probably familiar with these processes. For example, if you've ever been turned on, congratulations! You experienced endocrine signaling. Endocrine signaling is also at work any time you've felt stressed out from a difficult experience or a grueling task, or if you've felt anxiety from an impending deadline. A woman's menstrual cycle is also part of endocrine signaling. The hormones that signal the beginning and end of different phases of the menstrual cycle get their cues from this process.

Essential oils can help soothe or enhance the ups and downs of your endocrine system's natural processes. Whether you're trying to banish pain and stress or signal to your body that the time is ripe for a sensual romp, these essential oils are here to support you:

BASIL: Supports adrenal glands and boosts mood

BLACK PEPPER: Increases circulation, signals libido, eases anxiety

CEDARWOOD: Supports menstrual cycle, acts as a sedative, relieves stress

CHAMOMILE: Relaxes muscles, soothes menstrual cramps, relieves anxiety

CLARY SAGE: Anti-inflammatory, soothes PMS and menstrual cramps, tones uterus, supports thyroid

FRANKINCENSE: Relieves stress, supports thyroid, soothes menstrual cramps, tones uterus

GERANIUM: Relieves stress, boosts mood, eases menopausal symptoms

JASMINE: Soothes menstrual cramps, signals libido, tones uterus

LAVENDER: Relieves stress and anxiety, soothes menstrual cramps, tones uterus

MYRRH: Relieves stress, supports thyroid, soothes menstrual cramps, tones uterus

NEROLI: Relieves stress, soothes menopausal symptoms, signals libido

PATCHOULI: Relieves stress and anxiety, signals libido

PINE: Boosts mood and relieves stress and anxiety

ROSE: Relieves menstrual cramps, tones uterus, supports the menstrual cycle

ROSEMARY: Relieves stress and anxiety

SAGE: Relieves stress and anxiety

SANDALWOOD: Relaxes and calms, signals libido

SWEET MARJORAM: Supports the menstrual cycle, eases PMS and menstrual cramps, tones the uterus

YLANG-YLANG: Boosts mood, soothes PMS, signals libido

The right combinations of these essential oils can help calm anxiety and stress, soothe menstruation symptoms, support menstrual health, and encourage a healthy libido. Dilute them in a carrier oil or use them in a diffuser to support your endocrine system. Try some of these recipes to get you started.

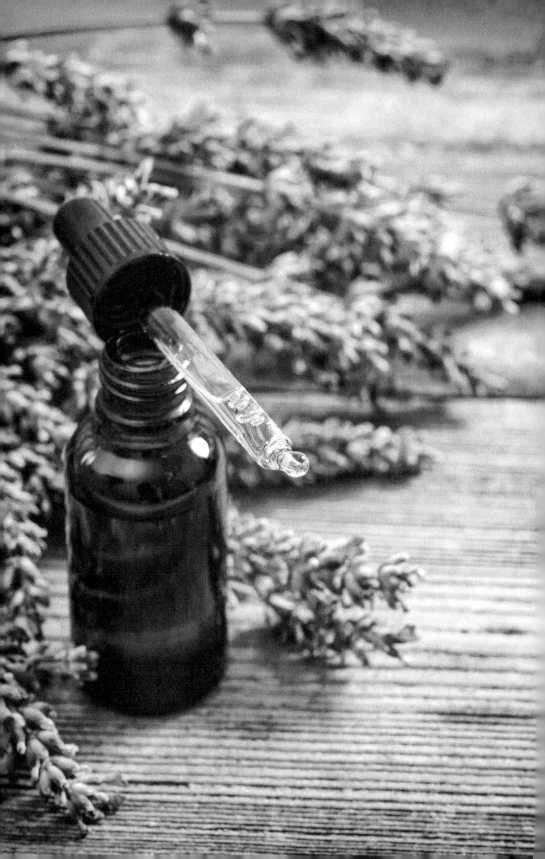

Blends for Endocrine Health

ANXIETY RELIEF BLEND

Anxiety can be draining. Tense muscles and a feeling of dread not only keep you from relaxing and sleeping well, but can also suck the pleasure and enjoyment out of everyday life. Anxiety is taxing to your adrenal glands and inspires them to overproduce cortisol. This can result in adrenal fatigue or adrenal exhaustion in extreme cases. Too much cortisol can overtax your system and burn you out. Lack of quality, uninterrupted sleep and stress don't just negatively affect cortisol levels, they also inspire your body to store more fat in the belly area and cause tiredness. Regular exercise and meditation can be beneficial in easing anxiety, and essential oils can add the right support to provide some relief. Breathe in this grounding Anxiety Relief Blend while you meditate to calm your mind and body.

> Lavender essential oil
>
> Chamomile essential oil
>
> Pine essential oil
>
> Cedarwood essential oil
>
> Sage essential oil
>
> Rosemary essential oil
>
> Basil essential oil

In your diffuser, combine 2 drops each of Lavender, Chamomile, Pine, Cedarwood, Sage, Rosemary, and Basil essential oils with the appropriate amount of water for your diffuser. Diffuse the oils into the air and inhale the calming aroma as you meditate. Afterwards, relax with a cup of lavender and chamomile tea to boost the calming effects.

MENSTRUAL CRAMP RELIEF RUB

Menstrual cramps are never fun. They can come on suddenly and can leave you in debilitating pain. Curl up with a hot water bottle and massage this Menstrual Cramp Relief Rub into your lower abdomen to help relieve the pain. This mix of floral essential oils will help soothe your pain and ease the stress and discomfort of menstruation. A bar of low-fat chocolate also couldn't hurt.

Sweet Marjoram essential oil

Clary Sage essential oil

Chamomile essential oil

Lavender essential oil

Jasmine essential oil

Rose essential oil

Carrier oil

Combine 2 drops each of Sweet Marjoram, Clary Sage, Chamomile, Lavender, Jasmine, and Rose essential oils with 1½ tablespoons of your favorite carrier oil, such as Jojoba, Coconut, or Sweet Almond oil. Mix to dilute the essential oils and massage a small amount into your lower abdomen above your uterus. Relax with a hot water bottle against your abdomen and a cup of raspberry leaf tea to help ease your pain.

SENSUAL OIL BLEND

The secret to a successful romantic encounter isn't in a special food or a secret potion: it's relaxing! Feeling relaxed and secure with your partner are keys to helping your romance blossom into fruition. This Sensual Oil Blend should help stir you in the right direction with its mix of mood-boosting, stress-busting, and libido-enhancing essential oils.

Ylang-ylang essential oil

Jasmine essential oil

Neroli essential oil

Lavender essential oil

Patchouli essential oil

Sandalwood essential oil

In your diffuser, combine 2 drops each of Ylang-ylang, Jasmine, Neroli, Lavender, Patchouli, and Sandalwood essential oils with the appropriate amount of water for your diffuser. Turn the diffuser on as you prepare for your date with your partner and breathe in the relaxing, uplifting scent of these floral oils. You'll leave smiling and in a sexy mood that's sure to rub off on your partner.

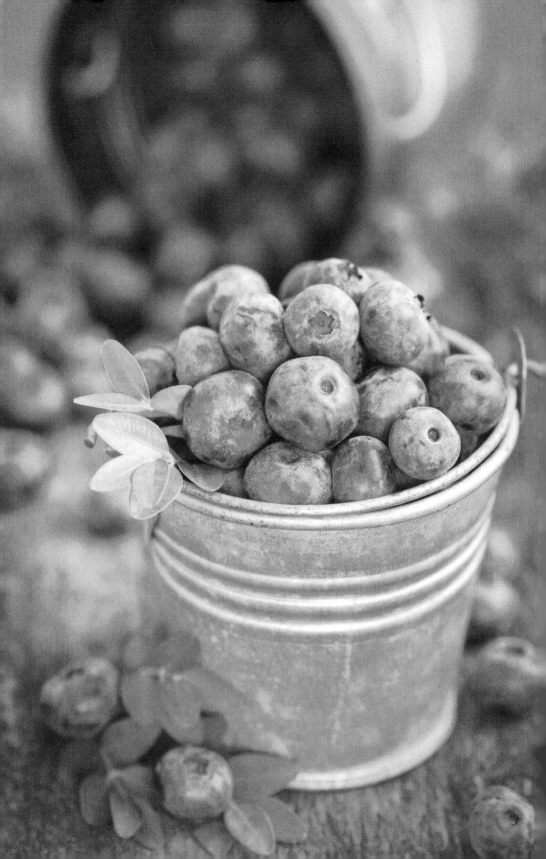

Chapter 11

Delicious Essential Oil Food and Beverage Recipes

"Gratitude unlocks the fullness of life. It turns what we have into enough, and more. It turns denial into acceptance, chaos to order, confusion to clarity. It can turn a meal into a feast, a house into a home, a stranger into a friend."

—Melody Beattie

We all know that essential oils are great for topical application, but did you know you can ingest them, too? Move aside, salt and pepper; stand out of the way, imitation lemon juice . . . the new sheriffs in town not only bring the flavor, they pack a pretty nice health punch, too! More and more health-conscious, holistic chefs are reaching for the essentials, and it's easy to see why.

When we integrate essential oils into our cooking, we open the door to greater health. Essential oils contain potent healing properties. By using them in cooking we have the opportunity to harness their healing properties in a more expansive way. It gives us the chance to consume essential oils on a regular basis, which is a boon to our vitality and well-being.

Essential oils provoke the body to initiate a self-healing sequence. If you ingest essential oils on a regular basis, you keep your body energized and in a continual mode of healing. By doing that, you don't give your energy a chance to stagnate. The same principles apply if you administer essential oils topically or diffuse them.

In this chapter we will enjoy some fun recipes that give us an opportunity to consume health promoting essential oils in our food and beverages.

BAKED TOMATO AND CHÈVRE DIP

Yield: 4 servings

This recipe is so simple, it borders on ridiculous. Mix, bake, serve, and enjoy the immune-boosting properties (courtesy of Oregano and Basil oils) just as much as the savory taste.

> 1 garlic clove, minced
>
> 3 tablespoons olive oil
>
> 2 cups cherry tomatoes, halved
>
> Sea salt and freshly ground black pepper
>
> 8–10 ounces goat cheese
>
> 2 drops Oregano oil
>
> 2 drops Basil oil
>
> Fresh oregano and basil
>
> Bread of choice

Preheat oven to 350°F.

Combine minced garlic, olive oil, halved tomatoes, and salt and pepper to taste.

Arrange mixture around the cheese in a medium baking dish and bake for 10–15 minutes (or until soft).

After removing the baking dish from the oven, extract 1 tablespoon of oil from the dish and mix with Oregano and Basil oils. Pour over cheese and tomatoes.

Garnish dish with fresh oregano and basil, and serve with bread.

CHÈVRE CRANBERRY DIP

Yield: 22 ounces

Revitalizing Lime, Orange, and Dill essential oils, paired with antioxidant-boosting cranberries, make this dish more than an indulgence—it's a health-enhancing bonanza!

    12 ounces cranberries

    1 bunch dill, chopped

    1 drop Dill essential oil

    8-10 ounces chèvre goat cheese

    ½ cup fresh lime juice

    1 drop Lime essential oil

    1 drop Sweet Orange essential oil

    ¼ teaspoon organic stevia powder (without fillers or dextrose)

Preheat oven to 350°F.

Chop and mix fresh cranberries, dill, and Dill essential oil.

Add lime juice, Lime and Orange essential oils, and stevia.

Stir in the goat cheese until combined, cover, and bake in a preheated oven for 20 minutes.

Serve with crackers, chips, or breads of your choice.

CINNAMON CLOVE LOW-CARB GRANOLA DESSERT BRUSCHETTA

Yield: 4 servings

This is a sweet, healthy treat that's sure to surprise kids and adults alike. So much crunch! And just a drop of Cinnamon and Clove oils goes a long way toward promoting dental health, alleviating pain, and balancing blood sugar.

    2 large apples

    ½ cup granola

    ½ cup unsweetened almond butter

    1 drop Cinnamon essential oil

    1 drop Clove essential oil

    Powdered cinnamon (optional)

Core apples and slice. Combine granola, almond butter, and oils. Spread granola mixture on apple slices and dig in! Sprinkle with powdered cinnamon for an extra, spicy kick, if desired.

CITRUS-DILL BALSAMIC VINAIGRETTE

Yield: 1 serving

Who needs store-bought dressing when you can whip up a healthy (and easy) alternative in two minutes flat? The essential oils in this vinaigrette infuse the tangy topping with immune-enhancing properties, so feel free to drizzle it on with abandon.

- 2 teaspoons balsamic vinegar (you can also make this with apple cider vinegar)
- 2 teaspoons Dijon mustard
- 2 teaspoons organic honey
- 4 drops Grapefruit essential oil, Lemon essential oil, and/or other citrus essential oils of your choice
- 4 tablespoons extra-virgin olive oil
- 1 tablespoon dried minced onion
- 1 teaspoon dried or fresh dill weed

Combine all ingredients and mix well.

Voilà! Add to salad or sauté with veggies.

CREAMY VEGAN SWEET POTATO BITES

Yield: 2 servings

Why use regular black pepper on sweet potato bites when you can use Black Pepper essential oil? It is a powerful antioxidant and aids digestion. Additionally, because it's antibacterial, you can power up your health while enjoying the decadent snack. Mixed with healthy fresh veggies, as well as detoxifying lemon and lime, this party snack will make guests forget their manners.

3 tablespoons olive oil, plus more for greasing the pans

1 drop Black Pepper essential oil

2 sweet potatoes, peeled

½ teaspoon Celtic sea salt

2 ripe avocados, mashed

2 drops Lemon oil

1 drop Lime oil

1 tablespoon fresh lime juice

1 clove garlic, minced

¼ teaspoon chili powder

¼ teaspoon paprika

2 tablespoons chopped fresh cilantro (optional)

2 diced Roma tomatoes, seeded (optional)

Salt and pepper to taste

Preheat oven to 425°F.

Line two baking sheets with foil and grease with olive oil. Blend Black Pepper oil and olive oil to taste. Slice sweet potatoes thinly, and place in a single layer on baking sheets.

Coat sweet potatoes with the mixture of olive oil and Black Pepper oil and add sea salt. Cook 20 minutes or until golden. Turn slices over and cook for 10–12 minutes more.

Remove from oven and cool. While cooling, combine avocados, essential oils, lime juice, garlic, and spices. Add avocado mixture to sweet potato slices and garnish with cilantro and tomatoes (if desired). Add salt and pepper to taste.

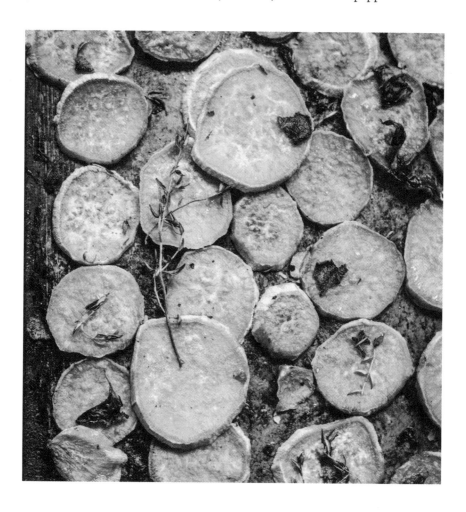

EDAMAME GUACAMOLE

Yield: About 4 servings

This guacamole serves up a protein and phytoestrogen punch, and delights the senses with flavor-enhancing essential oils. Not only do the citrus oils keep the guac from going gray, these antidepressant and antiseptic essentials put ordinary citrus liquids to shame.

> 2 cups frozen shelled edamame (thawed)
>
> 2 ripe avocados
>
> 2 drops Lemon essential oil
>
> 1 drop Lime essential oil
>
> 1 tablespoon lime juice
>
> 1 clove minced garlic
>
> 2 tablespoon onion (chopped)
>
> 1 large tomato (chopped)
>
> Salt and pepper to taste
>
> 4 tablespoons chopped cilantro (optional)

Purée edamame in a food processor on low speed. Peel and pit avocados and mash. Combine edamame and avocado, and fold together until well mixed.

Add essential oils, lime juice, garlic, onion, and tomatoes. Stir until mixed well, add salt and pepper to taste, and top with cilantro (if desired). Serve with tortilla chips, crackers, or dish of your choice!

FRUITY QUINOA TABBOULEH SALAD

Yield: 2 servings

This tabbouleh is crowned with a refreshing mélange of juices, oils, and spices. Lemon is a great stomach-calmer, while Grapefruit oil is a known stress-reliever.

- 1 cup quinoa, uncooked
- 1½ cups water
- Salt to taste
- 1 red grapefruit (peeled and chopped)
- 2 oranges (peeled and chopped)
- ⅔ cup chopped dried apricots
- ¼ cup pine nuts
- 1 cup fresh parsley

DRESSING

- 4 drops Lemon oil
- 4 drops Grapefruit oil
- 1 tablespoon olive oil
- 1 garlic clove, crushed
- 1 teaspoon paprika
- Pinch salt

Rinse quinoa. Place in a saucepan with water, simmer for 10 minutes (uncovered). Add salt and remove from the heat, covering until the quinoa is soft.

Remove from heat and add salt. Leave covered for 10 minutes until water is absorbed and grain is soft.

Combine chopped grapefruit, oranges, and apricots.

Combine ingredients for dressing. Add dressing and fruit to the quinoa and mix until combined. Garnish the quinoa with pine nuts and chopped herbs.

GINGER SPRING ROLLS WITH NUT SAUCE

Yield: 12 spring rolls

You wouldn't think one drop of Ginger essential oil would do much, but a drop is all you need to kick this tasty dish into eye-widening territory. Mixed into the cabbage, the ginger goes to work, infusing the rolls with uplifting, digestion-promoting deliciousness.

12 circular rice paper wrappers

¼ cup shredded red cabbage

1 drop Ginger essential oil

½ cup romaine lettuce

3 medium carrots, sliced into moderate sticks

½ cucumber, sliced into moderate sticks

½ cup mung bean sprouts

¼ cup basil leaves (chopped)

¼ cup cilantro leaves (chopped)

1 drop Lime essential oil

1 drop Cilantro essential oil

PEANUT SAUCE

3 tablespoons peanut butter (or almond butter)

1 tablespoon soy sauce

2 tablespoons maple syrup

4 tablespoons warm water

1 drop Lime essential oil

1 drop Cilantro essential oil

Peanuts or almonds (chopped)

For the Ginger Spring Rolls: Place each rice wrapper in a dish of warm water with one drop of Lime essential oil and one drop of Cilantro essential oil until soft. Remove from the water, and place on a damp kitchen towel (or a strong paper towel). Place the cabbage in a bowl and mix with the Ginger essential oil. Place lettuce on the rice paper and top with the remaining veggies and cabbage mixture. Wrap roll tightly, adding basil and cilantro as you go. Secure, and continue filling and rolling the remaining wraps.

For the Sauce: Combine all sauce ingredients in a blender and blend until creamy. Add water if the mixture is too thick. Remove from the blender and top with peanuts or almonds.

Dip Ginger Spring Rolls in the sauce and enjoy!

HONEY-GINGER LEMONADE

Yield: 4 servings

Forget the sugar-packed lemonades found in the grocery cases. This refreshing beverage is simple, quick, and, best of all, loaded with just enough Ginger essential oil to warm the body, mind, and soul.

    4 cups lemon juice

    ¼ cup lime juice

    ½ cup honey (or ½ teaspoon powdered stevia)

    5 drops Ginger essential oil

Mix citrus juices, sweetener, and essential oil in a tall glass pitcher. Add as much water as you think you need, stir, and taste until satisfied.

Place ice in a cup, pour, and enjoy!

KALE ORANGE SMOOTHIE

Yield: 4 servings

This delightful treat is chock-full of fruits and essential oils that make for an easy, enjoyable, mood-lifting system cleanse.

- 2 cups kale
- 2 cups frozen berries of your choice
- 1 cup frozen banana or pineapple
- 2 cups water or nut or rice milk
- 1–3 drops Sweet Orange essential oil
- Protein powder of your choice (optional)
- Organic honey (optional)

Mix or blend ingredients on high until thoroughly combined. Add protein powder, if desired.

Add a few drops of honey for added sweetness, if desired.

Enjoy chilled!

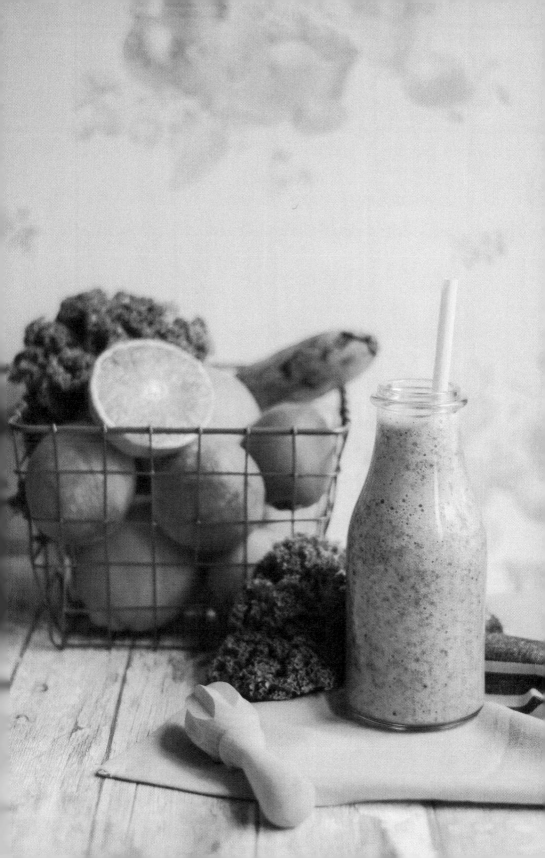

LAVENDER CUPCAKES WITH CHAMOMILE FROSTING

Yield: 1 dozen cupcakes

Cupcake shops had their 15 minutes of fame, but essential oil–infused cakes still await their moment in the limelight. One little drop goes a long way, and the Lavender/Chamomile combo is not only complementary, it's stress-relieving, too!

½ cup softened butter

¾ cup honey (or sweetener of choice)

2 large eggs

2 cups flour

2 teaspoons baking powder

½ teaspoon salt

1 cup low-fat milk or almond milk

6 drops Lavender essential oil

FROSTING

4 ounces softened cream cheese

2 teaspoons pure vanilla extract

2 ounces butter

6 drops Chamomile essential oil

5 cups confectioners' sugar

Orange zest (optional)

Sprinkles (optional)

Edible flowers (optional)

For the cupcakes: Preheat oven to 375°F and line muffin tin with muffin cups. Beat butter, Lavender essential oil, and honey until fluffy, then add one egg at a time and mix until combined. Mix flour, baking powder, and salt, and add to the butter mixture.

Pour milk slowly into the batter, mixing as you pour. Fill muffin tins and bake for 18–20 minutes. Allow cupcakes to cool before frosting them.

For the frosting: Beat cream cheese, vanilla extract, butter, and essential oil until creamy. Add sugar slowly while beating, continuing to beat until the mixture is fluffy and free of lumps. Frost the cupcakes, garnish with orange zest, sprinkles, and/or edible flowers (if desired) and serve!

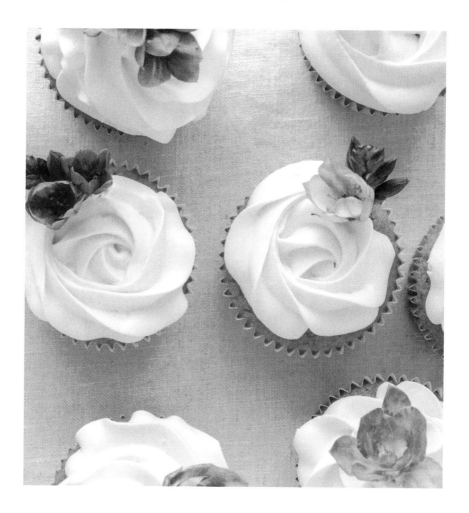

LEMON ESSENTIAL OIL YOGURT

Yield: 2 servings

A few drops of Lemon essential oil transforms yogurt from "blah" to "ah!" Give your digestive flora and fauna a one-two punch with this powerful probiotic delight.

  1½ cups plain yogurt (goat, sheep, coconut, or regular)

  2 teaspoons lemon juice

  3 drops Lemon essential oil

  10 drops liquid stevia (or honey)

  1 tablespoon slivered almonds

Mix yogurt, lemon juice, essential oil, and sweetener until combined.

Add more sweetener or essential oil, if needed.

Top with almonds and dig in!

LOW-SUGAR, GLUTEN-FREE, BLUEBERRY-LEMON MUFFINS

Yield: 12 muffins

The words *sugar-free* and *gluten-free* may ease our minds (and bellies!), but our taste buds may rear back in fear. Worry not, because these creations are out-of-this-world tasty. A healthy kick of Lemon oil tantalizes the tongue while breaking down fat, boosting energy, and improving digestion.

  2 cups gluten-free flour

  1 teaspoon xanthan gum

  1 tablespoon baking powder

  ½ teaspoon salt

  ½ cup brown rice syrup

  8 drops Lemon oil

  1 egg or 1 tablespoon applesauce

  1 cup coconut, almond, or rice milk

  ½ cup butter (or ghee or vegan margarine), melted

  1 cup blueberries, fresh or frozen

Combine dry ingredients.

Combine wet ingredients and stir into the dry mixture.

Add blueberries.

Divide the mixture among 12 muffin cups.

Bake for 20–25 minutes at 375°F.

Serve warm with a dollop of butter and honey for sweetness!

MINTY STRAWBERRY-ALMOND SALAD WITH RASPBERRY-LIME DRESSING

Yield: 4 servings

This sweet salad pairs well with quinoa or rice. You can enjoy the vinaigrette on various dishes, or stick to splashing it on fresh, immune-enhancing spinach and antioxidant-boosting berries.

RASPBERRY VINAIGRETTE:

2 cups raspberries

4 drops Lime essential oil

¼ cup olive oil

1 tablespoon honey (or sweetener of choice)

2 tablespoons mustard powder

2 tablespoons lime juice

SALAD:

10 ounces baby spinach or romaine lettuce

2 cups sliced strawberries

½ cup slivered almonds

½ cup diced cucumbers

½ cup chickpeas

¼ cup fresh chopped mint

½ cup feta cheese (optional)

For the vinaigrette: Mash raspberries in a bowl. Whisk in oils, sweetener, mustard powder, and lime juice until combined. Chill for 30 minutes in refrigerator.

For the salad: Combine all salad ingredients. Splash vinaigrette onto the salad and enjoy cold!

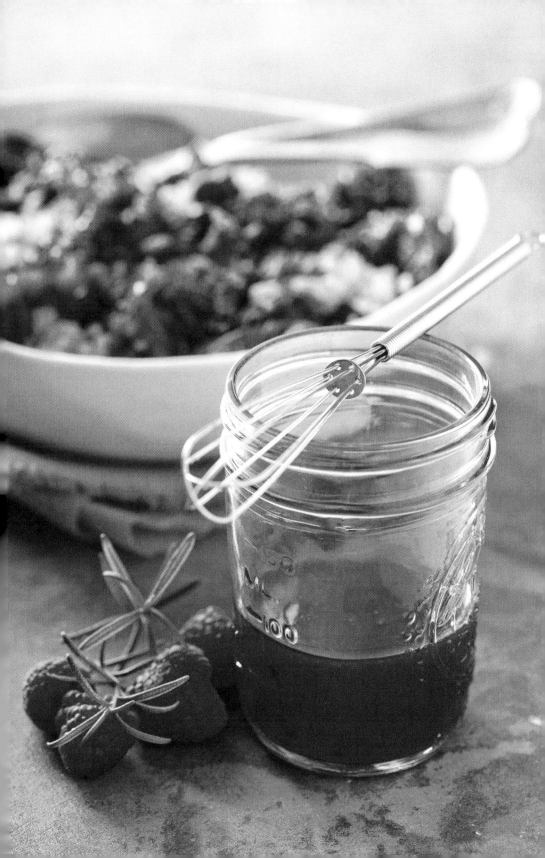

RAINBOW ORANGE FRUIT PARFAIT

Yield: 1 serving

Toss into a bowl whatever fruit you have lying around, spray with whipped cream, and enjoy the invigorating blast of citrus that'll leave you smelling like a sun-kissed orange grove.

Fruit of choice (the more colorful, the better!)

2 drops Orange essential oil

1 cup whipped cream

Cut fruit into bite-size pieces of equal proportion. Mix in essential oil.

Place ¼ of the fruit mixture in a glass cup, add a layer of cream on top, add another ¼ of the fruit mixture, top with another layer of cream, and repeat until your cup is filled. Place in the refrigerator for 30 minutes (for extra refreshment) and enjoy!

RASPBERRY-LEMON YOGURT PANCAKES

Yield: 2 servings

Whip these up, toss on some fresh raspberries for added flavor and vitamin C, and enjoy the sweet satisfaction of having your pancakes and eating them, too. The Lemon oil in these flapjacks will infuse you with more energy than a double espresso (with no crash and burn) to boot.

1¾ cups all-purpose flour

1 tablespoon baking powder

3 tablespoons granulated sugar or a pinch of stevia powder

¼ teaspoon kosher salt

2 large eggs

2–3 drops Lemon essential oil

2 tablespoons olive oil

⅔ cup plain, sheep, or Greek yogurt

⅔ cup almond or coconut milk

1 teaspoon vanilla extract

1 cup raspberries

Maple syrup, butter/ghee, berries of choice

Whisk dry ingredients together and set aside.

Whisk wet ingredients together until combined. Add the dry ingredients to the wet mixture and stir until just combined. Add raspberries and stir once more.

Drop mixture onto a greased, heated griddle or skillet.

Cook for 3 minutes, or until golden brown on one side, then flip and repeat. Top with syrup, butter, berries, or other toppings of your choice.

SLOW-COOKED VEGAN BEANS

Yield: 3 servings

Easy peasy pinto beans! Toss the ingredients into slow cooker and wait in anticipation for the citrusy lime and fresh cilantro aromas to waft through the house. A splash of alkalizing apple cider vinegar, a plethora of antioxidant-rich fresh veggies, and a dash of tangy spices make this a go-to meal for the dreaded summer sniffles.

- 2 cups pinto beans, black soy beans, or black beans, uncooked
- 4 tablespoons cumin
- 3 teaspoons paprika
- 2 tablespoons garlic flakes
- 2 tablespoons garlic, minced
- ½ teaspoon chili powder
- ½ teaspoon paprika
- 1 small onion, minced
- 2 tomatoes, diced
- 1½ cups fresh arugula or spinach, chopped
- 5 cups water
- 2 tablespoons coconut oil
- 2 cups apple cider vinegar or lime juice
- 1–2 drops Cilantro oil
- 1–2 drops Lime oil

Wash beans and soak them overnight.

Place the beans in a slow cooker, adding the dry ingredients and the spices.

Add minced onions and garlic.

Add diced tomatoes and arugula or spinach.

Add water, coconut oil, apple cider vinegar, and Cilantro oil until pot is full. Stir until combined.

Cover and cook on High 4–6 hours.

Add Lime oil and serve!

STRAWBERRY-ROSE VANILLA POPS

Yield: 6–12 pops (depending on the size of your molds)

If you're looking for a lighter alternative to ice cream, set your sights on these easy-to-make pops. You can't go wrong with crushed pineapple and Rose essential oil (especially in the romance and self-love departments!).

- 32 ounces vanilla yogurt
- 20 ounces finely chopped fresh strawberries
- 6 drops Rose essential oil

Mix ingredients until combined. Fill popsicle molds. Freeze for 4–6 hours, and enjoy!

VEGAN BLUEBERRY-LAVENDER ICE CREAM

Yield: 4 servings

Ice cream is the perfect treat for end-of-summer festivities, and this recipe is of the guilt-free variety. The blueberries pack an antioxidant punch, the coconut cream adds healthy fats, and the Lavender oil infuses the sweet dessert with a delightful floral taste.

2 cups frozen blueberries

1 cup coconut cream

1 tablespoon Blue Agave oil

4 drops Lavender oil

⅓ cup coconut water

⅛ cup unsweetened coconut flakes

Place parchment or wax paper on a large dish or container.

Mix blueberries, coconut cream, and essential oils in a blender.

Slowly add coconut water while continuing to blend.

Drop mixture in a freezer-safe bowl, cover securely, and place in the freezer for a few hours (or overnight).

Top with coconut flakes.

Once firm, enjoy the ice cream in a bowl or a cone!

WARM ROSEMARY-LEMON CASHEWS

Yield: 2 cups

If you could assign the word *comfort* to a taste, rosemary would be the sure-fire winner. This heartwarming, belly-filling dish includes a nice dose of nutty protein and a splash of powerful antioxidants.

    16 ounces cashews

    2 tablespoons olive oil

    Lemon zest

    3 sprigs rosemary

    4 drops Rosemary essential oil

    2 drops Lemon essential oil

    ¾ teaspoon sea salt

Place nuts on a baking sheet and roast for 10 minutes at 375°F until golden brown. Simmer olive oil, lemon zest, and rosemary on the stove. Add roasted cashews, and stir until coated. Remove from heat, add essential oils, and top with a pinch of salt. Enjoy warm.

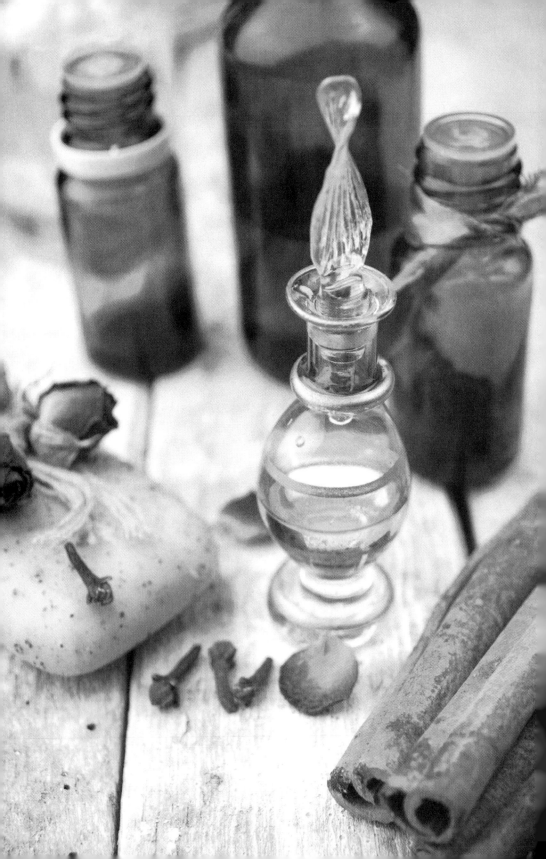

Chapter 12

Rejuvenating At-Home Spa Recipes with Essential Oils

"It's a good idea always to do something relaxing prior to making an important decision in your life."

—Paulo Coelho

Self-care is an essential part of a healthy life. Making the daily commitment to treating yourself with the kindness, respect, and regard you would offer to a cherished friend or family member is essential for your emotional and mental health. We all know that stress is a huge culprit behind many diseases and ailments and that self-care is the first course of action in reducing stress. Plus, it feels good. When you sink into a relaxing home spa treatment you allow yourself to let go of thinking and doing. You also give yourself a powerful dose of self-love because you are communicating via a concrete action that you are worth the time and effort it takes to relax and recharge. A simple home spa treatment can be a powerful healing force in your life.

Essential oils figure in many at-home remedies to smooth the skin, soothe the spirit, and calm the mind. The following recipes offer a plethora of benefits from simple combinations of these wonderful oils.

ACNE-FIGHTING FACIAL WASH

Acne happens to the best of us, no matter how old we are. Essential oils are the best tools for healing those unsightly blemishes. Frankincense and Tea Tree essential oils are especially powerful for treating acne. They both have strong antiseptic qualities, particularly Tea Tree essential oil. Lavender essential oil helps to soothe irritated skin blemishes and promote healing, while a carrier oil like Grape Seed or Almond oil moisturizes skin. Altogether, this Acne-Fighting Facial Wash packs a powerful punch and will help you fight and recover from blemishes with regular use.

Distilled water

Grape Seed or Almond oil

UNSCENTED LIQUID CASTILE SOAP: All-natural, chemical-free soap

VITAMIN E OIL: Improves skin moisture and elasticity

FRANKINCENSE ESSENTIAL OIL: Antiseptic, astringent, lifts and tightens skin

TEA TREE ESSENTIAL OIL: Antiseptic, soothes dry skin

LAVENDER ESSENTIAL OIL: Soothes skin irritations, promotes healing

Combine ¼ cup Unscented Liquid Castile Soap, ¼ cup distilled water, 2 teaspoons either Grape Seed oil or Almond oil, 1 teaspoon vitamin E oil, and 3 drops each of Frankincense, Tea Tree, and Lavender essential oils. Store in a bottle with a pump lid and shake to combine. Use 1–2 squirts to gently cleanse your face with your hands or a washcloth. Rinse well and follow with your preferred toner and moisturizer.

BRIGHTENING TURMERIC FACE MASK

Dull, tired, or irritated skin gets some TLC with the Brightening Turmeric Face Mask. Turmeric is a natural anti-inflammatory and works wonders to calm irritated skin and acne while drawing out a healthy glow. Lemon essential oil supports turmeric by cleansing toxins from the skin to improve your complexion and leave skin soft and bright. Raw organic honey brings it all together to moisturize and heal any wounds or irritations. With regular use of this mask, you'll be left with glowing, calm skin and a radiant complexion.

TURMERIC POWDER: Anti-inflammatory, calms irritated skin and acne

RAW ORGANIC HONEY: Antibacterial, moisturizes, heals wounds

LEMON ESSENTIAL OIL: Improves complexion, softens skin, cleanses toxins

Combine ½ teaspoon turmeric powder, 1 tablespoon raw organic honey, and 1–2 drops Lemon essential oil. Wash your face first to remove any makeup or dirt. Smooth the mask over your face, being careful to avoid the eye area. Leave the mask on for 15 to 20 minutes, and then rinse. If you have any leftovers, cover and store them in the refrigerator. Use twice a week for best results.

CALMING BODY WASH

Gently cleanse your skin and recover from a rough day with this Calming Body Wash. Lavender essential oil supplies vital antioxidants and combines with Chamomile essential oil to relieve stress and anxiety, and ease any skin irritations. Give your skin a gentle scrub with this body wash and feel your stress slip away.

UNSCENTED LIQUID CASTILE SOAP: All-natural, chemical-free soap

RAW ORGANIC HONEY: Antibacterial, moisturizes, heals wounds

JOJOBA OIL: Soothes and moisturizes skin, noncomedogenic

VITAMIN E OIL: Improves skin moisture and elasticity

LAVENDER ESSENTIAL OIL: Antioxidant, relieves anxiety, reduces skin irritation, promotes healing

CHAMOMILE ESSENTIAL OIL: Relieves anxiety, anti-inflammatory, reduces skin irritation

In a mixing bowl, combine ⅔ cup Unscented Liquid Castile Soap, ¼ cup raw organic honey, 2 teaspoons Jojoba oil, 1 teaspoon vitamin E oil, and 15 drops each Lavender and Chamomile essential oils. Mix until well incorporated, being careful not to create suds from the soap. Store in an 8-ounce bottle in your shower.

CINNAMON CACAO BODY SCRUB

Indulge your senses and wake up your skin with this sweet Cinnamon Cacao Body Scrub. Cinnamon essential oil increases your circulation, warming up your skin in the process. It might also give your libido a healthy spike. Ground cacao nibs and coarse sugar exfoliate your skin, while raw organic honey and coconut oil moisturize. You'll step out of the shower feeling pampered and energized for your day.

COARSE SUGAR: Exfoliates

GROUND CACAO NIBS: Exfoliate

RAW ORGANIC HONEY: Antibacterial, moisturizes

COCONUT OIL: Skin moisturizer

CINNAMON ESSENTIAL OIL: Increases circulation, stimulates libido

In a mixing bowl, combine ½ a cup coarse sugar, ¼ cup ground cacao nibs, ¼ cup raw organic honey, 2 tablespoons Coconut oil, and 7 drops Cinnamon essential oil. Use a spoon to combine the ingredients and store in an airtight jar. Scrub your skin before your shower, being careful to avoid sensitive areas or mucous membranes.

CITRUS BATH BOMBS

Bath bombs are a fizzy treat, and with a homemade recipe you can have an endless supply. These Citrus Bath Bombs will brighten your mood and leave your skin feeling reinvigorated and smooth. Lemon, Orange, and Grapefruit essential oils all work to relieve stress, soften skin, improve your complexion, and kill bacteria, while the additional bath bomb ingredients soften and hydrate your skin. Pop one of these in the tub, and you'll be feeling bright and cheery inside and out.

Citric acid

Bath bomb mold or muffin tin

BAKING SODA: Softens skin

EPSOM SALT: Magnesium-rich, reduces pain and inflammation

ORGANIC CORNSTARCH: Softens skin and soothes irritation

COCONUT OIL: Hydrates skin

ORANGE ESSENTIAL OIL: Improves complexion, antibacterial, relieves stress

LEMON ESSENTIAL OIL: Improves complexion, softens skin, cleanses toxins

GRAPEFRUIT ESSENTIAL OIL: Increases circulation, antibacterial, antifungal, relieves stress

Combine the dry ingredients (8 ounces baking soda, 4 ounces citric acid, 4 ounces Epsom salt, 4 ounces organic cornstarch) in one bowl and the liquid ingredients (2 tablespoons heated Coconut oil, Citric acid 3 teaspoons water, 10 drops each Orange, Lemon, and Grapefruit essential oils) in a separate bowl. Add the liquid ingredients to the dry ingredients a few drops at a time, mixing well with your hands. Feel free to wear gloves to reduce the mess or protect sensitive skin. When all the ingredients are combined, the mixture should hold together without crumbling when squeezed in your fist. Add a little more water if it still hasn't reached this stage. From here, grease your bath bomb mold with more Coconut oil and firmly pack the mixture in. Let the bath bombs sit for 24–48 hours or until dry. Then, remove the bath bombs from the molds and store them in an airtight bag. Use within two weeks.

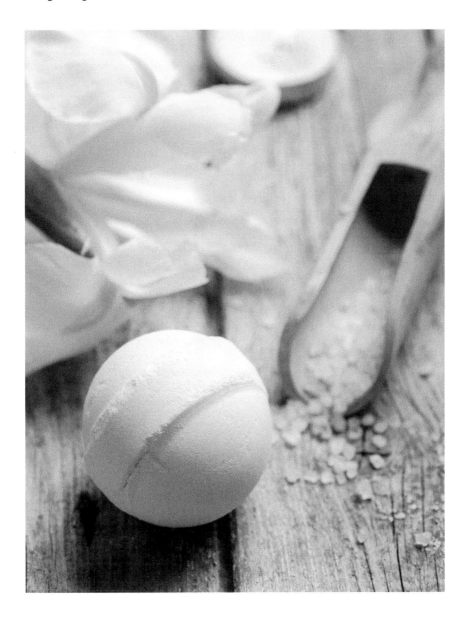

CLEANSING GRAPEFRUIT SCRUB

Grapefruit essential oil is the star of this fruity pink body scrub. It promotes blood flow circulation and acts a stress reliever while also providing antibacterial and antifungal benefits for your skin. Try it out in the morning for an extra boost to your day.

HIMALAYAN SEA SALT: Exfoliates skin and provides color

COCONUT OIL: Hydrates skin

GRAPEFRUIT ESSENTIAL OIL: Increases circulation, relieves stress, antibacterial, antifungal

In a mixing bowl, combine half a cup of Himalayan sea salt, 2 tablespoons of Coconut oil, and 10 drops of Grapefruit essential oil. Mix the ingredients together with a spoon and place the mixture in an airtight jar. Before your shower, scrub your body down with this delicious-smelling pink salt to brighten your mood and leave your skin silky-soft.

EVENING BODY WASH

A rough day at work increases stress levels and can make it difficult to get to sleep. Wash away the day's difficulties with this relaxing Evening Body Wash. Frankincense and Bergamot essential oils relieve stress and anxiety, and Lavender essential oil boosts your mood and improves your sleep quality. Bergamot essential oil also acts as a sedative, putting you in the mood to slip under the covers and get some rest.

UNSCENTED LIQUID CASTILE SOAP: All-natural, chemical-free soap

RAW ORGANIC HONEY: Antibacterial, moisturizes, heals wounds

JOJOBA OIL: Soothes and moisturizes skin, noncomedogenic

VITAMIN E OIL: Improves skin moisture and elasticity

LAVENDER ESSENTIAL OIL: Relieves stress and anxiety, boosts mood, improves sleep

FRANKINCENSE ESSENTIAL OIL: Relieves stress and anxiety

BERGAMOT ESSENTIAL OIL: Relieves stress, sedative

In a mixing bowl, combine ⅔ cup Unscented Liquid Castile Soap, ¼ cup raw organic honey, 2 teaspoons Jojoba oil, 1 teaspoon vitamin E oil, and 10 drops each Lavender, Frankincense, and Bergamot essential oils. Mix until well incorporated, being careful not to create suds from the soap. Store in an 8-ounce bottle in your shower. Use in the evening or whenever you need to relax.

REJUVENATING BODY SCRUB

If you're feeling a little down or under the weather, this Invigorating Body Scrub is sure to kick up your mood. Ginger, Black Pepper, and Cinnamon essential oils combine to pump you up and bring your mojo back. Together they increase your circulation, reduce muscle or headache pain, provide relief from anxiety, and work to stimulate your libido. They also provide a delicious warming sensation that's sure to shake you out of your funk.

BROWN SUGAR: Exfoliates skin

GINGER ESSENTIAL OIL: Anti-inflammatory, warming, relieves anxiety

BLACK PEPPER ESSENTIAL OIL: Warming, reduces muscle pain

CINNAMON ESSENTIAL OIL: Increases circulation, stimulates libido

RAW GINGER ROOT: Powerful antioxidant, anti-inflammatory, warming (optional)

Combine 1 cup brown sugar with 10 drops each Ginger, Black Pepper, and Cinnamon essential oils. If you want an extra boost, chop an ounce of fresh gingerroot and put it in the food processor until it reaches a pastelike consistency. Mix all ingredients together and place in an airtight jar. Before your shower, scrub your skin with this mixture and enjoy the invigorating warmth. Avoid mucous membranes or any sensitive areas.

INVIGORATING HAIR AND SCALP MASK

Give your hair and scalp a pick-me-up with this Invigorating Hair and Scalp Mask. Rosemary essential oil stimulates your scalp to strengthen and support hair growth, while Peppermint essential oil works as an antiseptic to treat dry skin. Nutrient-rich avocado and hydrating Coconut oil combine to moisturize both hair and scalp and boost shine. You'll be sporting luscious locks after regular use of this mask.

AVOCADO: Moisturizes scalp and hair, adds shine to hair

COCONUT OIL: Moisturizes scalp and hair

ROSEMARY ESSENTIAL OIL: Stimulates and improves hair growth

PEPPERMINT ESSENTIAL OIL: Stimulates scalp, antiseptic

Combine 1 avocado (peeled and pitted), 2 tablespoons Coconut oil, and 5 drops each Rosemary and Peppermint essential oils in a blender. Pour into a bowl and apply to hair and scalp. Let sit for 15–20 minutes and rinse well. Use regularly once a week for stronger and shinier hair.

MORNING CITRUS BODY WASH

Sometimes it's a little difficult to wake up in the morning. Wash away drowsiness with some Morning Citrus Body Wash. Lemon, Orange, and Grapefruit essential oils all work to relieve stress, soften and improve your complexion, and kill bacteria. They are also proven to boost your mood and relieve any stress and anxiety, making them the perfect wake-up call.

UNSCENTED LIQUID CASTILE SOAP: All-natural, chemical-free soap

RAW ORGANIC HONEY: Antibacterial, moisturizes, heals wounds

JOJOBA OIL: Soothes and moisturizes skin, noncomedogenic

VITAMIN E OIL: Improves skin moisture and elasticity

LEMON ESSENTIAL OIL: Improves complexion, softens skin, cleanses toxins, boosts mood

ORANGE ESSENTIAL OIL: Improves complexion, antibacterial, relieves anxiety

GRAPEFRUIT ESSENTIAL OIL: Increases circulation, antibacterial, antifungal, relieves stress

In a mixing bowl, combine ⅔ cup Unscented Liquid Castile Soap, ¼ cup raw organic honey, 2 teaspoons Jojoba oil, 1 teaspoon vitamin E oil, and 10 drops each Lemon, Orange, and Grapefruit essential oils. Mix until well incorporated, being careful not to create suds from the soap. Store in an 8-ounce bottle in your shower. Use in the morning or whenever you need a boost to your mood.

NIGHTTIME BATH OIL

Unwind and prepare your mind and body for sleep with this Nighttime Bath Oil. Lavender essential oil calms and eases tension in your body and mind, while earthy Cedarwood essential oil produces serotonin to relax and release melatonin, the sleep hormone produced by the pineal gland. Frankincense essential oil reduces stress and anxiety to set the stage for a balanced mood the following morning, and Bergamot essential oil relieves any nervous tension to produce a calming feeling. Light some candles and soak a while in this warm, soothing bath to ease your way into restful sleep.

JOJOBA OIL: Soothes and moisturizes skin, noncomedogenic

LAVENDER ESSENTIAL OIL: Relieves stress and anxiety, boosts mood, improves sleep

CEDARWOOD ESSENTIAL OIL: Encourages serotonin production, anti-inflammatory, relieves stress

FRANKINCENSE ESSENTIAL OIL: Relieves stress and anxiety

BERGAMOT ESSENTIAL OIL: Relieves stress, sedative

Combine 1 tablespoon Jojoba oil with 4 drops each Lavender, Cedarwood, Frankincense, and Bergamot essential oils. Add to your bath and rub any floating oil bubbles into your skin. Relax and let the soothing scent lull you toward sleep.

OIL-REDUCING CLAY MASK

Oily skin can be overwhelming. So this Oil-Reducing Clay Mask, combined with a gentle cleanser that does not completely strip all of the natural oils from your face, can help manage your skin. Bergamot essential oil is a superstar in this area, as it cleanses and tones oily skin. Combined with bentonite clay, this mask will help soak up your excess oil while soothing and cleansing your skin in the process.

> Water
>
> BENTONITE CLAY: Draws out bacteria, oils, and toxins, soothes irritation
>
> BERGAMOT ESSENTIAL OIL: Cleanses and tones oily skin, antibacterial

In a small bowl, combine 1 tablespoon bentonite clay, 1–2 tablespoons water, and 4 drops Bergamot essential oil. Mix until it forms a spreadable paste and apply to your face with your fingers or a brush. Be careful to avoid the eye area. Leave the mask on for 10–15 minutes, and then rinse. Use up to twice a week for best results.

POST-WORKOUT EUCALYPTUS BATH SALTS

After pushing your body to the limit at the gym, a relaxing soak in the tub is just what you need to relieve those sore muscles. These Eucalyptus Bath Salts will help you rest and recover from your favorite workout. The Eucalyptus and Peppermint essential oils work together with Epsom salts to reduce inflammation and relax tight, sore muscles. As a bonus, the refreshing scent will open your sinuses and help you breathe more easily.

EPSOM SALT: Magnesium-rich, reduces pain and inflammation

EUCALYPTUS ESSENTIAL OIL: Powerful anti-inflammatory

PEPPERMINT ESSENTIAL OIL: Relaxes tight muscles, relieves pain

JOJOBA ESSENTIAL OIL (OPTIONAL): Soothes and moisturizes skin, noncomedogenic, supports healing

In a mixing bowl, combine 2 cups Epsom salt with 30 drops Eucalyptus essential oil and 10 drops Peppermint essential oil. If you want to soften your skin in the process, add a ¼ cup of Jojoba oil as well. Mix to combine and store in an airtight jar. Add a ¼ cup to your warm bathwater and soak away your aches and pains.

RELAXING MASSAGE OIL

A soothing massage can help relieve the stress of a difficult day and nourish both mind and body. This Relaxing Massage Oil utilizes Frankincense and Myrrh essential oils to relieve stress and anxiety. Frankincense essential oil acts as an astringent and has anti-inflammatory properties to soothe any aches or pains, while Myrrh essential oil alleviates skin irritations, moisturizes, and has antibacterial and antifungal properties to keep your skin healthy. Rub away the stress on your own or with a partner and enjoy this timeless aroma.

> JOJOBA OIL: Soothes and moisturizes skin, noncomedogenic
>
> MYRRH ESSENTIAL OIL: Soothes skin irritations, moisturizes, antibacterial, antifungal, relieves stress
>
> FRANKINCENSE ESSENTIAL OIL: Relieves stress and anxiety, astringent, anti-inflammatory

Combine 1 ounce of Jojoba oil with 6 drops each Myrrh and Frankincense essential oils. Store in a dark-colored container.

ROSEMARY-EUCALYPTUS BATH BOMBS

After a vigorous workout, it's important to relax and take care of your body. Pop a Rosemary Eucalyptus Bath Bomb into your tub and soak away any aches or pains. Rosemary and Eucalyptus essential oils both contain strong anti-inflammatory properties to soothe your sore muscles. Your body will thank you in the morning!

Water

BAKING SODA: Softens skin

CITRIC ACID: Adds fizz

EPSOM SALT: Magnesium-rich, reduces pain and inflammation

ORGANIC CORNSTARCH: Softens skin and soothes irritation

HEATED COCONUT OIL: Hydrates skin

ROSEMARY ESSENTIAL OIL: Anti-inflammatory

EUCALYPTUS ESSENTIAL OIL: Anti-inflammatory

BATH BOMB MOLD OR MUFFIN TIN

Combine the dry ingredients (8 ounces baking soda, 4 ounces citric acid, 4 ounces Epsom salt, 4 ounces organic cornstarch) in one bowl and the liquid ingredients (2 tablespoons Coconut oil, 3 teaspoons water, 15 drops each Rosemary and Eucalyptus essential oils) in a separate bowl. Add the liquid ingredients to the dry ingredients a few drops at a time, mixing well with your hands. Feel free to wear gloves to reduce the mess or protect sensitive skin. When all the ingredients are combined, the mixture should hold together without crumbling when squeezed in your fist. Add a little more water if it still hasn't reached this stage. From here, grease your bath bomb mold with more Coconut oil and firmly pack the mixture in. Let the bath bombs sit for 24–48 hours or until dry. Then, remove the bath bombs from the molds and store them in an airtight bag. Use within two weeks.

ROSEMARY-PEPPERMINT SEA SALT HAIR SPRAY

Gently tousled beach waves seem to be all the rage. Up your style game and nourish your hair and scalp at the same time with this Rosemary-Peppermint Sea Salt Hair Spray. Rosemary and Peppermint essential oils not only create a delightful scent for your hair but also stimulate hair growth and act as an antiseptic. You'll be rocking beachy waves and some healthy hair as well.

EPSOM SALT: Adds texture to hair

SEA SALT: Stiffens hold

ALOE VERA GEL: Provides hold, moisturizes

ROSEMARY ESSENTIAL OIL: Stimulates and improves hair growth

PEPPERMINT ESSENTIAL OIL: Stimulates scalp, antiseptic

Combine 1 cup hot but not boiling water with 2 tablespoons Epsom salt, ½ teaspoon sea salt, 1 teaspoon aloe vera gel, and 4 drops each Rosemary and Peppermint essential oils. Mix until the salts are dissolved and pour into a spray bottle. Spray onto damp hair and scrunch for loose, beachy waves, or spray onto dry hair at the roots for volume. Store at room temperature for three to four months.

ROSE MILK BATH

There is nothing more luxurious than roses. A creamy Rose Milk Bath is the ultimate indulgence you can treat your skin to. Rose essential oil has been used in natural beauty compounds for centuries. It increases your skin's permeability, allowing you to absorb more nutrients. Geranium essential oil, in turn, reduces inflammation and supports cell growth. Together they balance hormones and work to soothe your skin. When you're finished luxuriating in this bath, you'll have silky-smooth skin, fit for a queen.

POWDERED WHOLE MILK: Moisturizes skin

ORGANIC CORNSTARCH: Softens skin and soothes irritation

BAKING SODA: Softens skin

ROSE ESSENTIAL OIL: Increases skin permeability, balances hormones, antibacterial

GERANIUM ESSENTIAL OIL: Reduces inflammation, balances hormones, supports cell growth

Mix 2 cups powdered whole milk, ½ cup organic cornstarch, ½ cup baking soda, and 5 drops each Rose and Geranium essential oils. Mix and store in an airtight jar. Pour 1 cup of this powder under hot, running bathwater and treat yourself to this sweetly scented bath. Feel free to substitute powdered coconut milk for a vegan option.

SENSUAL BATH OIL

Scent can set the mood, and if you're looking to get lucky with your date, some Sensual Bath Oil can tip the scales in your favor. Ylang-ylang, Jasmine, and Patchouli essential oils all stimulate the libido and work to relieve stress and anxiety. You'll approach your date feeling calm, confident, and sexy, and the scent of your skin will have your partner feeling the vibe.

JOJOBA OIL: Soothes and moisturizes skin, noncomedogenic

YLANG-YLANG ESSENTIAL OIL: Boosts libido, boosts mood, relieves inflammation,

JASMINE ESSENTIAL OIL: Boosts libido, relieves stress and anxiety

PATCHOULI ESSENTIAL OIL: Boosts libido, regenerates skin cells, relieves anxiety

Combine 2 tablespoons of Jojoba oil with 3 drops each of Ylang-ylang, Jasmine, and Patchouli essential oils. Add to your bath and rub any floating oil bubbles into your skin. Soak in the sensual scents and give yourself that extra boost to ensure a successful date night.

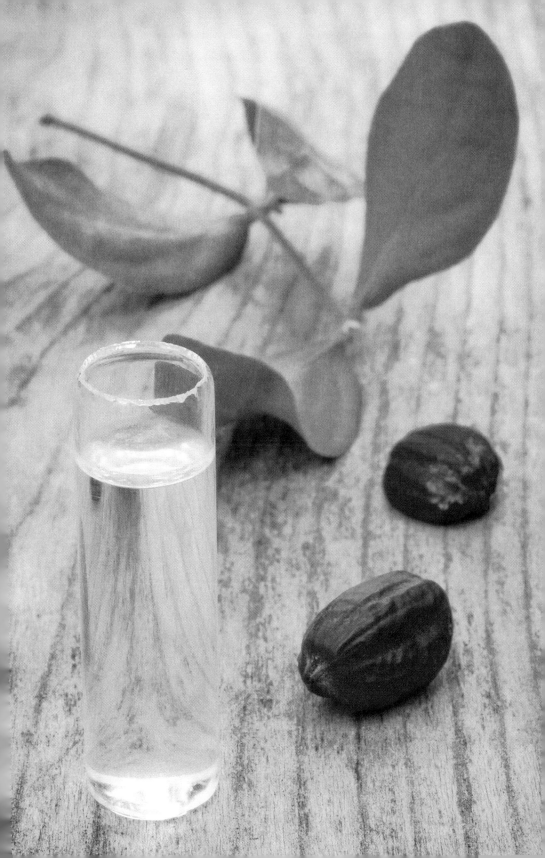

CALMING ROSE AND HONEY FACE MASK

Dry, irritated skin can be a hassle. Renew and replenish with a Soothing Rose and Honey Face Mask. Rose essential oil increases your skin's permeability, allowing it to absorb more nutrients and become more hydrated. With regular use, this sweet mask will leave your face looking plump and healthy.

RAW ORGANIC HONEY: Antibacterial, moisturizes

ALMOND OIL: Moisturizes skin

ROSE ESSENTIAL OIL: Increases skin permeability, balances hormones, antibacterial

Combine 2 tablespoons raw organic honey, 1 tablespoon Almond oil, and 5 drops Rose essential oil. Massage into your face after cleansing, avoiding the eye area, and let it rest for 15–20 minutes. Rinse well and continue with your preferred toner and moisturizer. Store any leftovers, covered, in the refrigerator. Use twice a week for best results.

SOOTHING WINTER BATH OIL

Dry winter air is a recipe for cracked, irritated skin. Recover from trudging through snow and ice by taking a dip in this Soothing Winter Bath Oil. The combined Lavender, Neroli, and Geranium essential oils will soothe your chapped skin and quicken the healing process, while the floral scent should boost your spirits.

JOJOBA OIL: Soothes and moisturizes skin, noncomedogenic, supports healing

LAVENDER ESSENTIAL OIL: Soothes skin irritations

NEROLI ESSENTIAL OIL: Regenerates skin, improves elasticity, has antioxidant properties

GERANIUM ESSENTIAL OIL: Speeds healing, anti-inflammatory

Combine 1 tablespoon Jojoba oil with 5 drops Lavender essential oil, 5 drops Neroli essential oil, and 5 drops Geranium essential oil. Add to your bath and rub any floating oil bubbles into your skin. Relax and enjoy the sweet, floral scent while winter winds blow outside.

VANILLA ROSE SUGAR SCRUB

This Vanilla Rose Sugar Scrub is surely the sweetest way to exfoliate and pamper your skin. Rose essential oil makes your skin more permeable so it can absorb more nutrients and moisture from the scrub. It also is antibacterial and hormone balancing. You'll walk out of your bathroom with smooth and supple skin, smelling of sweet vanilla and roses.

BROWN SUGAR: Exfoliates

ROSE ESSENTIAL OIL: Increases skin permeability, balances hormones, antibacterial

VANILLA EXTRACT: Fragrance, boosts mood

RAW ORGANIC HONEY: Antibacterial, moisturizes

In a bowl, combine 1 cup brown sugar with 30 drops Rose essential oil, 1 teaspoon vanilla extract, and ¼ cup raw organic honey. Mix all ingredients together and place the mixture in an airtight jar. Before your bath or shower, scrub your skin and enjoy the delicious scent. Avoid mucous membranes or any sensitive areas.

WARMING MASSAGE OIL

Massage is not just a great way to relax or a sexy buildup to a romp with a partner. It can also heal and strengthen sore and aching muscles. The right massage oil can help boost the healing process for sore or tight muscles. Use some Warming Massage Oil next time your calves tighten up. The warming and anti-inflammatory effects of Ginger and Black Pepper essential oils will relax those taut muscles and ease away any pain.

JOJOBA OIL: Soothes and moisturizes skin, noncomedogenic

GINGER ESSENTIAL OIL: Anti-inflammatory, warming, relieves anxiety

BLACK PEPPER ESSENTIAL OIL: Warming, reduces muscle pains

Combine 1 ounce of Jojoba oil with 6 drops each of Ginger and Black Pepper essential oils. Store in a dark-colored container.

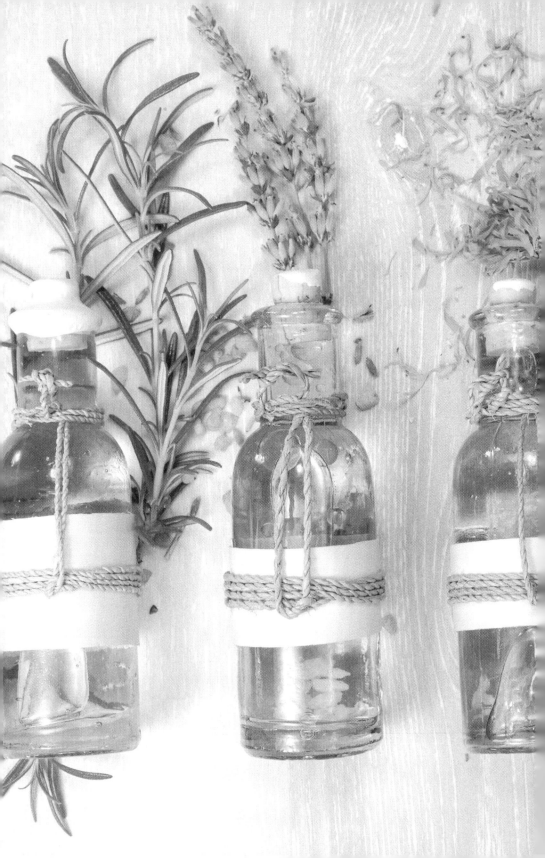

Frequently Asked Questions

There is a lot of information out there about essential oils. Some of it is good and useful, some not so much. In this section, I've compiled the most frequently asked questions and answered them. Here is a summary of the information that will allow you to use essential oils confidently and safely to improve your life.

How much essential oil is helpful and safe to consume orally in one day?

* For adults, it's ideal to consume between 2 and 4 drops a day. You should never consume more than 24 drops in any one day.

* For children, it's ideal to consume 1 to 2 drops a day. Children should never consume more than 12 drops in any one day. Children under the age of two should not consume essential oils orally at all.

* In the case of essential oils, more is not better. You should start at the lowest possible dose and work your way up from that.

How much essential oil is helpful and safe to consume topically in one day?

* For adults, it's ideal to consume between 3 and 6 drops a day. You should never consume more than 36 drops in any one day.

* For children, it's ideal to consume 1 to 2 drops a day. Children should never consume more than 12 drops in any one day. Essential oils should not be used on children under the age of 6 months. Use only in a diffuser for children between 6 months and 2 years old. From 2 years until the age of 12 years, essential oils can be applied topically as long as they are used in concentrations not exceeding 1 percent.

* When using essential oils, it is particularly important to keep an eye on the concentration of oils that you are using. All the essential oils, except for Lavender and Tea Tree oils, should be diluted to a concentration of no more than 3 percent to prevent irritation and burns.

* Some oils, such as Cinnamon, can cause irritation when applied topically. If you find that the essential oil is irritating your skin, reduce the concentration to no more than 1 percent or stop using the oil completely.

How much essential oil is helpful and safe to consume through inhalation in one day?

You have a lot more latitude when it comes to essential oils that are inhaled. There are no set maximums here, but it does pay to use common sense. For most therapeutic purposes, around half an hour of exposure to the essential oils will be more than sufficient. Use as needed.

Of course, your symptoms will dictate how long you diffuse the oils. If you have a head cold, for example, you might want to diffuse the oils for a few hours to help clear up the congestion and keep your sinuses clear. If, on the other hand, you need a boost to get you going in the morning, a few whiffs of the oil might be all you need.

It should also be said that you can develop a tolerance for essential oils over time and this makes them less effective. It is better to start off with the lowest possible dose and work your way up from there.

Is it better to use only therapeutic grade oils?

Yes, it is actually crucial to use only therapeutic grade oils. There is a huge difference between therapeutic grade oils and the so-called scent oils. The latter are usually synthetic and, though they may smell the same, they have none of the beneficial compounds found in essential oils.

Therapeutic grade oils are 100 percent pure and naturally based. Scent oils are not. They are likely to have harmful compounds in them as well.

Is it better to use only organic essential oils?

* It is beneficial to choose organic essential oils only because of the extraction process used.

* Some oils, such as Jasmine, will not stand up to the process of heat extraction and so need a gentler extraction method. Solvent extraction is a less expensive and gentler means of extracting the oils, but it does mean that traces of the solvent are left in the oils themselves.

* You also do not want to consume harmful pesticides. And organic farming is much better for the earth!

Are essential oils still as healthy to consume when they are cooked?

* People sometimes worry that when they're used in cooking, essential oils will either evaporate or undergo changes to their chemical structures that may render them unsafe. You can minimize the risks of either by adding essential oils as late as you possibly can in the cooking process. That said, however, studies have found that some essential oils stand up to boiling temperatures rather well.

* It is extremely important, if you are using essential oils in cooking, to use top-quality, therapeutic grade oils.

Is a carrier oil used when rubbing essential oils on your skin?

* Essential oils are highly concentrated, so there is a risk of chemical burns or irritation if they are applied directly to the skin. As the oils do not disperse in water, you need to mix them with a carrier oil in order to dilute them.

* A carrier oil is quite simply a dilution agent for your essential oils. You can, however, choose carrier oils based on their beneficial properties as well.

What are the best types of carrier oils?

* Sweet Almond oil is one of the most popular oils, as it works with all skin types and is fairly light. It is especially beneficial for those with dry skin. It is stable and has a long shelf life.

* Grape Seed oil is also suitable for most skin types and is also light. It is slightly astringent and so better suited to those with normal/oily skin. It is stable and has a long shelf life.

* Coconut oil is another option. It is great for smoothing and moisturizing the skin and can be used for your hair as well. It should be noted, however, that Coconut oil can cause sensitivity over an extended period, so stop using it if you start to develop a rash.

* There are many other carrier oils that are beneficial but these three are the best.

Which carrier oils are the least likely to clog your pores?

Arian oil, Calendula oil, Sweet Almond oil, Hemp Seed oil, Avocado oil, Emu oil, Baobob oil, Neem oil, Borage oil, Rose Hip Seed oil, Evening Primrose oil, Grape Seed oil, Jojoba oil, Peach Kernel oil.

How can you use essential oils for cleaning?

Add a few drops of oil to the rinse water when cleaning off your counters, the bathtub, etc. You can also add a few drops to the final rinse cycle when you're doing laundry. Place a few drops into the vacuum bag when vacuuming to lightly scent your home.

How many calories are in a few drops of most essential oils?

The caloric content of a few drops of essential oils is negligible.

What nutrients are in a few drops of essential oils?

The contents of the oil itself depend on which oil you choose. That said, the nutrient content is low because of the quantity consumed.

However, some nutrients are trace minerals to begin with and they may be beneficially absorbed.

How much sugar and carbohydrates are in orally consumed essential oils?
Again, this is negligible, so, yes, you can use essential oils if you are on a low-carb diet.

What studies have been conducted on the health-related benefits of essential oils?

* Antibiotic/antimicrobial effect: Researchers have shown a renewed interest in essential oils as a means of combating antibiotic-resistant infections. Tea Tree oil and Eucalyptus oil have been proved to be as effective as standard treatments for staph infections.

* Depression, anxiety, and stress: Studies have centered mainly on Lavender oil, and there is evidence that lavender helps reduce anxiety when used in a dentist's waiting room and that it can assist in calming patients who suffer from dementia. Studies on Clary Sage have proven that it has an antidepressant effect.

* Digestive system: While drinking a cup of peppermint tea may prove useful in settling an upset stomach, studies have shown that the essential oils, taken internally, are a lot more useful. The studies measured usefulness when the oils were ingested in enteric-coated tablets. These tablets protect the oil from the stomach acid and allows it to pass to the gut for the treatment of irritable bowel syndrome.

How many times a day is optimal to ingest essential oils for different ailments?
This depends on the nature of the ailment and the symptoms you have. For example, if you are taking an oil to treat the flu, it makes sense to take some of the oil every four hours or so to give symptomatic relief.

It is best to start at the lowest dose possible and increase it, if necessary.

Divide the dose equally over the number of waking hours for conditions like cold and flu, and depression. For conditions like insomnia, take the oil around about half an hour or an hour before bedtime.

How many times a day is optimal to topically apply essential oils for different ailments?
Again, this depends on what symptoms you are treating. For skin conditions, such as eczema, it is advisable to apply the oils three to four times a day. For fungal infections, like ringworm, the oils should be applied around five to six times a day.

Another option is to apply the oils topically as necessary. When you have sore muscles, for example, you would usually only need to apply the oils once or twice.

Are essential oils safe for children?
This depends on how old the children are.

* Children 6 months or younger should not be exposed to essential oils because of the oils' strong detoxifying effects. Sensitization to the oils may also occur during this period.

* From 6 to 12 months, you can start to use the oils in a diffuser. Check that the oils are child-safe before using them.

* Once children are 2 years old, you can start applying the oils topically. This might mean a drop of oil in the bath or a topically applied oil diluted to a concentration of no more than 1 percent.

What essential oils cannot be used by pregnant women?
In the case of essential oils during pregnancy, it is better to be safe than sorry. Using the wrong oils could lead to high blood pressure, uterine contractions, and/or miscarriage.

* The gentler oils, such as Lavender and Chamomile, are safe bets to use when you're pregnant.

* Some oils, such as Geranium oil, should be avoided during the first trimester of pregnancy but can be used after that. For safety's sake, avoid using any oils besides Lavender and Chamomile at all during the first trimester.

* Essential oils should not be taken internally at all during pregnancy and the oils that you are using topically should be diluted to a concentration of no more than 1 percent of the total mixture.

* The following oils should not be used during any stage of pregnancy: Blue Cypress, Carrot Seed, Cinnamon Bark, Clary Sage, Dill, Fennel, Hyssop, Tansy, Jasmine, Lemongrass, Lemon Myrtle, Marjoram, Melissa, Myrrh, Nutmeg, Ravintsara, Rosemary, Sage, and Wintergreen.

What essential oils can be used by nursing women?

* When nursing, you need to use a lower concentration of essential oils. Keep the oils diluted to no more than 1 percent concentration. An easy way to work this out is that for every tablespoon of carrier oil, add 1 to 2 drops of the essential oil.

* When applying the oils, don't use them close to the breasts within an hour before the baby feeds.

* When nursing, do not take essential oils internally unless you're under a health care professional's care.

* Oils to promote milk supply: Clary Sage, Basil, and Fennel will promote milk supply. Use the oils for no more than 10 days at a time and then give it a break for at least 3 or 4 days.

* Oils to promote calm: Lavender, Bergamot, Neroli, Rose, and Geranium oils are all good for promoting calm.

* Oils for alleviating stretch marks: Lavender, Neroli, Geranium, and Sandalwood are good when diluted in Sweet Almond oil. Boost the healing effects even more by adding 10 percent of either Rose Hip oil or Calendula oil.

EPILOGUE

I hope you have enjoyed our odyssey through the fascinating world of essential oils, exploring the many ways they can heal the body, mind, and spirit naturally without harsh chemicals and side effects.

In a world of endocrine disrupting and ecologically irresponsible chemical use, we have the opportunity to choose products that are holistically healthy for our families and the planet. Essential oils are an indispensable part of that plan.

Everything we use on our bodies or in our homes goes somewhere. For instance, when you clean your sink with a typical chemical cleaner you are washing that product down the drain and eventually it will end up in the water supply. All of the water on Earth is ultimately connected through weather and geography.

Alternatively, you could choose a delightful and effective natural cleaning blend including essential oils and cause zero negative environmental impact through that choice. Plus, save your respiratory system from inhaling toxic fumes that aromatize with hot water as you are scrubbing and enter your system intradermally through your hands. Natural products for home and health are a win-win for you and the planet. So, scent your home and life with holistic superstars like essential oils and enjoy a light and aromatic existence full of vitality and joy!

GLOSSARY

ACUPRESSURE: A healing therapy in which pressure is applied to various parts of the body; essentially, acupuncture without the incorporation of needles.

ACUPUNCTURE: A type of alternative medicine, which originated in ancient China, in which fine needles are inserted into the body at numerous points in order to treat pain or other conditions.

AROMATHERAPY: The science of utilizing essential oils to enhance bodily functions.

CARRIER OIL: An oil with either very little or no scent that is used as a dilution agent for essential oils.

DETOXIFY: The process by which toxic properties are removed from the body.

DISTILLATION: A process of separating liquid substances through boiling.

ESSENTIAL OILS: Highly concentrated and deliciously aromatic compounds that have been pressed or distilled from plants.

DIFFUSERS: Devices that disperse essential oils into the air everywhere from an office to a bedroom.

HOT EFFLEURAGE: A method of oil extraction.

HYDROSOL: The scented water extracted from oils by hot effleurage.

PATCH TEST: A method of testing a small area of skin with a substance to determine if any irritation occurs.

REFLEXOLOGY: A massage process aimed to treat bodily issues, with special focus on reflex points.

WARMING OIL: Oil that helps to speed blood circulation.

METRIC CONVERSION CHART

U.S. SYSTEM	METRIC SYSTEM
Volume	
1 teaspoon	5 mL
1 tablespoon	15 mL
¼ cup	60 mL
½ cup	120 mL
¾ cup	175 mL
1 cup	240 mL
Mass	
1 ounce	28 grams
4 ounces	110 grams
8 ounces	224 grams
12 ounces	340 grams
16 ounces	455 grams
Temperature	
300°F	150°C
325°F	160°C
350°F	180°C
375°F	190°C
400°F	200°C
425°F	220°C
450°F	230°C

Resources

BRANDS WE RECOMMEND

This is a list of the best quality essential oil brands:
* Oshadhi: only organic offerings recommended
* Simplers Botanicals
* Snow Lotus
* Veriditas Botanicals: organic, therapeutic, very high quality

BOOKS

Bell, Kristen Leigh. *Holistic Aromatherapy for Animals: A Comprehensive Guide to the Use of Essential Oils & Hydrosols with Animals* (Findhorn Press, 2002).

Bowles, E. Joy. *The Chemistry of Aromatherapeutic Oils* (Allen & Unwin, 2004).

Catty, Suzanne. *Hydrosols: The Next Aromatherapy* (Healing Arts Press, 2001).

Cunningham, Scott. *Magical Aromatherapy: The Power of Scent* (Llewellyn, 1998).

Davis, Patricia. *Subtle Aromatherapy* (Random House UK, 1996).

Lembo, Margaret Ann. *The Essential Guide to Aromatherapy and Vibrational Healing* (Llewellyn, 2016).

Schnaubelt, Kurt. *Medical Aromatherapy: Healing with Essential Oils* (Frog Books, 1998).

Schnaubelt, Kurt. *Advanced Aromatherapy: The Science of Essential Oil Therapy* (Healing Arts Press, 1998).

Worwood, Valerie Ann. *Aromatherapy for the Soul: Healing the Spirit with Fragrance and Essential Oils* (New World Library, 2006).

Worwood, Valerie Ann. *Aromatherapy for the Healthy Child: More Than 300 Natural, Nontoxic, and Fragrant Essential Oil Blends* (New World Library, 2000).

WEBSITES

For reputable and informative online resources about essential oils, check these websites:
* WEIL: www.drweil.com
* Acupuncture Today: www.acupuncturetoday.com
* The Amanda Apothecary: www.anandaapothecary.com/learn-archive

ACKNOWLEDGMENTS

I am eternally grateful to my kind and wonderful literally agent, Lisa Hagan. She is the catalyst that enables each literary journey in my life. I am so fortunate to work with the team at Sterling. They are a bevy of consummate professionals, especially Chris Barsanti, who has wisely guided this book to its gorgeous result with finesse and expertise, Lori Paximadis, and Diana Drew, who did a superb job copyediting the book. Talented designer Christine Heun produced stunning visuals for the project.

The delightful Karen Nino worked tirelessly to help me bring my dreams to life. I am forever grateful to my most steadfast supporters, my friends and family. Eight years ago, Dr. Laurie Nadel opened the doors to my writing career with her kindness and I am eternally thankful. Last but not least, you the reader are my reason for continuing to put proverbial pen to paper. May your days be joyfully bright and your evenings be perfumed with exotic jasmine night blooms and serene lavender blossoms.

PICTURE CREDITS

BIBLIOGRAPHY

WEBSITES

"A List of Non-Comedogenic Facial Oils." *The Best Organic Skin Care*. Accessed August 6, 2017. https://thebestorganicskincare.com/a-list-of-non-comedogenic-facial-oils.

"Antimicrobial efficacy of eucalyptus oil and 1, 8-cineole alone and in combination with chlorhexidine digluconate against microorganisms grown in planktonic and biofilm cultures. *Journal of Antimicrobial Chemotherapy*|"Oxford Academic." OUP Academic. https://academic.oup.com/jac/article/64/6/1219/743860/Antimicrobial-efficacy-of-eucalyptus-oil-and-1-8.

"*Aromatherapy Bible*." Aromatherapy Bible. http://aromatherapybible.com.

"Benefits and Uses of Niaouli Essential Oil." *Healthy and Natural World*. Accessed April 5, 2017.

"Bergamot Oil for Cleansing, Confidence & Body Cures." *Dr. Axe, Food Is Medicine*. Accessed August 6, 2017. https://draxe.com/bergamot-oil/.

"Chamomile Essential Oil." *Aromatherapy Bible*. http://aromatherapybible.com/chamomile/.

"Cinnamon Oil: 10 Proven Benefits and Uses." *Dr. Axe, Food Is Medicine*. Accessed May 22, 2017. https://draxe.com/cinnamon-oil/.

"Differences Between Essential Oil Grades." http://www.thelittleessentials.com/differences-between-essential-oil-grades/.

"DoTERRA Essential Oils." *Essential Oils Pure and Natural*. Accessed April 6, 2017. https://www.doterra.com/.

"DoTERRA Essential oils for Breastfeeding." *Healing in Our Homes*. Accessed April 12, 2017. https://healinginourhomes.com/essential-oils-and-breastfeeding/.

"11 Amazing Benefits of Cardamom." *Organic Facts*. Accessed August 6, 2017. https://www.organicfacts.net/health-benefits/herbs-and-spices/health-benefits-of-cardamom.html.

"Epsom Salt—The Magnesium-Rich, Detoxifying Pain Reliever." *Dr. Axe, Food Is Medicine*. Accessed April 5, 2017. https://draxe.com/epsom-salt/.

"Essential Oil." *Encyclopaedia Britannica*. Accessed August 8, 2017. https://www.britannica.com/topic/essential-oil.

"Essential Oil." *New World Encyclopedia*. Accessed August 27 2017. http://www.newworldencyclopedia.org/entry/Essential_oil.

"Essential Oil Pops." *Goodness Gathering*. http://goodnessgathering.blogspot.com/2014/06/essential-oil-pops.html.

"Essential Oil Reference Chart for Your Mind and Emotions." Aromatherapy Blog. Accessed July 28, 2017. http://www.thearomablog.com/reference-chart-essential-oils-mind/.

"*Essential Oils and Children*." *Using Essential Oils Safely*. Accessed August 6, 2017. http://www.usingeossafely.com/essential-oils-and-children/.

"Essential Oils for Allergies." *Natural Living Ideas*. Accessed May 1, 2017. http://www.naturallivingideas.com/essential-oils-for-allergies/.

"Essential Oils for Allergy Relief." *Healthy and Natural World*. Accessed August 9, 2017.

"Essential Oils Might Be the New Antibiotics." *The Atlantic*. Accessed May 17, 2017. https://www.theatlantic.com/health/archive/2015/01/the-new-antibiotics-might-be-essential-oils/384247/.

"Essential Oils That are Safe During Pregnancy and Nursing." *There's an EO For That*. Accessed July 14, 2017. http://www.theresaneoforthat.com/essential-oils-that-are-safe-during-pregnancy-and-nursing/.

"5 Essential Oils To Banish Brain Fog Once And For All." *Mindbodygreen.* Accessed April 6, 2017. https://www.mindbodygreen.com/0-25695/5-essential-oils-to-banish-brain-fog-once-and-for-all.html.

"15 Geranium Oil Benefits for Healthy Skin and Much More." *Dr. Axe, Food Is Medicine.* Accessed August 6, 2017. https://draxe.com/10-geranium-oils-benefits-healthy-skin-much/.

"Frankincense Essential Oil Uses and Benefits." *Healthy and Natural World.* 2017. Accessed May 4, 2017. http://www.healthyandnaturalworld.com/frankincense-essential-oil-uses-and-benefits/.

"Gattefossé's burn." *Robert Tisserand.* http://roberttisserand.com/2011/04/gattefosses-burn/. Accessed August 6, 2017.

"Geranium Essential Oil." *Aromatherapy Bible.* Accessed May 8, 2017. http://aromatherapybible.com/geranium/.

"Grapeseed Oil—Is It Healthy or Not?" *Dr. Axe, Food Is Medicine.* Accessed August 6, 2017. https://draxe.com/grapeseed-oil/.

"Guard-oil." *doTerra.* Accessed May 6, 2017. https://doterra.com/US/en/p/on-guard-oil.

"Gut-Friendly Ginger Essential Oil—Reduces Inflammation & Nausea." *Dr. Axe, Food Is Medicine.* Accessed April 2, 2017. https://draxe.com/ginger-essential-oil/.

"Health Benefits of Parsley." Organic Facts. Accessed May 28, 2017. https://www.organicfacts.net/health-benefits/herbs-and-spices/health-benefits-of-parsley.html.

"Health Benefits of Ravensara Essential Oil." *Organic Facts.* June 19, 2017. https://www.organicfacts.net/health-benefits/essential-oils/health-benefits-of-ravensara-essential-oil.html.

"Herbal Oil: Palmarosa Oil Benefits and Uses." Mercola.com. Accessed May 16, 2017. articles.mercola.com/herbal-oils/palmarosa-oil.aspx.

"Herbal Oil: Vetiver Oil Benefits and Uses." Mercola.com. Accessed July 6, 2017. http://articles.mercola.com/herbal-oils/vetiver-oil.aspx.

"History." *Essential Oil Academy.* http://essentialoilsacademy.com/history/.

"History Basics." *Alliance of International Aromatherapists.* Accessed August 6, 2017. http://www.alliance-aromatherapists.org/history-basics.

"History of Aromatherapy." *Quinessence Aromatherapy.* Accessed April 8, 2017. http://www.quinessence.com/history-of-aromatherapy.

"How to Buy Essential Oils." *Aroma Web.* Accessed July 16, 2017. https://www.aromaweb.com/articles/howtobuyessentialoils.asp.

"How Essential Oils Are Extracted." National Association for Holistic Aromatherapy.org. Accessed May 6, 2017. https://naha.org/explore-aromatherapy/about-aromatherapy/how-are-essential-oils-extracted/.

"How to Use Essential Oils for Allergies." *Organic Authority.* Accessed May 9, 2017. http://www.organicauthority.com/how-to-use-essential-oils-for-allergies/.

"Human Digestive System," *Encyclopaedia Britannica.* Accessed April 7, 2017. https://www.britannica.com/science/human-digestive-system/Secretions#ref212903.

"Human Endocrine System," *Encyclopaedia Britannica.* Accessed April 18, 2017. https://www.britannica.com/science/human-endocrine-system.

"Is it safe to use essential oils while I'm pregnant?" *BabyCentre UK.* Accessed May 17, 2017. https://www.babycentre.co.uk/x536449/is-it-safe-to-use-essential-oils-while-im-pregnant.

"Jasmine: Its Story in Aromatherapy." *Tim Noonan Consultant Speaker Coach.* Accessed May 6, 2017. https://timnoonan.com.au/resources/health-and-wellbeing/jasmine-story-aromatherapy/.

"Jasmine Oil—Mood Booster and Stress Buster." *Dr. Axe, Food Is Medicine.* Accessed August 6, 2017. https://draxe.com/jasmine-oil/.

Jojoba Oil—Skin and Hair Healer and Moisturizer." *Dr. Axe, Food Is Medicine.* Accessed April 6, 2017.https://draxe.com/jojoba-oil/.

"Lavender Cupcakes with Orange Frosting." *Growing Up Gabel.* Accessed July 22, 2017. https://growingupgabel.com/lavender-cupcakes-orange-buttercream-frosting.

"Melatonin and Sleep," National Sleep Foundation. Accessed May 27, 2017. https://sleepfoundation.org/sleep-topics/melatonin-and-sleep.

"Orange Oil—Enhance Your Immunity, Skin and Kitchen!" *Dr. Axe, Food Is Medicine.* Accessed August 6, 2017. https://draxe.com/orange-oil/.

"Pink Himalayan Salt Benefits that Make it Superior to Table Salt." *Dr. Axe, Food Is Medicine.* Accessed April 22, 2017. https://draxe.com/pink-himalayan-salt/.

"Rapid Actions of Xenoestrogens Disrupt Normal Estrogenic Signaling." *Steroids.* Accessed August 6, 2017. https://www.ncbi.nlm.nih.gov/pmc/articles/PMC3947648/.

Reduce Depression & Inflammation with Patchouli Oil." *Dr. Axe, Food Is Medicine.* Accessed May 6, 2017. https://draxe.com/patchouli-oil/.

"Roman Chamomile—Essential Oil Benefits & Uses." *Dr. Axe, Food Is Medicine.* Accessed July 26, 2017. https://draxe.com/roman-chamomile-essential-oil/.

"Rose Essential Oil." *Aromatherapy Bible.* Accessed May 24, 2017.http://aromatherapybible.com/rose/.

"Rose Essential Oil Benefits Skin, Depression, and Hormones." *Dr. Axe, Food Is Medicine.* Accessed May 25, 2017. https://draxe.com/rose-essential-oil-benefits-skin-depression-hormones/.

"Rosemary Oil Uses and Benefits." *Dr. Axe, Food Is Medicine.* Accessed April 7, 2017. https://draxe.com/rosemary-oil-uses-benefits/.

"Safe to Ingest Essential Oils Therapeutic vs. Food Grade." *Superfoodly.* Accessed May 6, 2017. https://www.superfoodly.com/safe-to-ingest-essential-oils-therapeutic-vs-food-grade/.

"Sandalwood Essential Oil." *Aromatherapy Bible.* Accessed July 5, 2017.http://aromatherapybible.com/sandalwood/.

"7 Lavender Oil Benefits for Healing." *Dr. Axe, Food Is Medicine.* Accessed July 8, 2017. https://draxe.com/lavender-oil-benefits/.

"16 Amazing Benefits of Cilantro or Corriander." *Organic Facts.* Accessed April 26, 2017.https://www.organicfacts.net/health-benefits/herbs-and-spices/health-benefits-of-coriander.html.

"Surviving Seasonal Allergies Using Essential Oils." *Diffuser World. Accessed April 26, 2017.* https://www.diffuserworld.com/FeedItem/Surviving-Seasonal-Allergies-Using-Essential-Oils/.

"10 Black Pepper Essential Oil Benefits You Won't Believe," *Dr. Axe, Food Is Medicine.* Accessed May 11, 2017. https://draxe.com/black-pepper-essential-oil/.

"*10 Geranium Oil Benefits for Healthy Skin and More.*" *Dr. Axe.* Accessed May 7, 2017. https://draxe.com/10-geranium-oils-benefits-healthy-skin-much/.

10 Proven Bentonite Clay Benefits and Uses," *Dr. Axe, Food is Medicine.* Accessed April 16, 2017. https://draxe.com/10-bentonite-clay-benefits-uses/.

"10 Proven Myrrh Oil Benefits and Uses," *Dr. Axe, Food Is Medicine.* Accessed July 7, 2017. https://draxe.com/myrrh-oil/.

"The impact of cooking and delivery modes of thymol and carvacrol on retention and bioaccessibility in starchy foods." *Food chemistry.* Accessed May 8, 2017. https://www.ncbi.nlm.nih.gov/pubmed/26593564.

"The Top 5 Allergy fighters." *Dr axe.* Accessed May 8, 2017.https://draxe.com/the-top-5-natural-allergy-fighters/.

"The Truth About Phototoxic Essential Oils & How To Use Them Safely." *Herbal Academy.* Accessed August 6, 2017. https://theherbalacademy.com/truth-phototoxic-essential-oils-use-safely/.

"13 Grapefruit Essential Oil Benefits—Starting With Weight Loss." *Dr. Axe, Food Is Medicine.* Accessed May 11, 2017.https://draxe.com/grapefruit-essential-oil/.

"13 Uses for Castile Soap—Natural Cleaning for Body and Home." *Dr. Axe, Food Is Medicine.* Accessed August 6, 2017. https://draxe.com/castile-soap/.

Thyme Essential Oil." *Young Living.* Accessed July 26, 2017.https://www.youngliving.com/en_EU/products/thyme-essential-oil.

"This Anxiety-Fighting Oil Primes Your Brain to Better Deal with Stress." *Dr. Axe.* Accessed May 11, 2017. https://draxe.com/vetiver-oil/.

"Top 10 Eucalyptus Oil Uses and Benefits." *Dr. Axe, Food Is Medicine.* Accessed April 16, 2017. https://draxe.com/eucalyptus-oil-uses-benefits/.

"Top 10 Lemon Essential Oil Uses and Benefits." *Dr. Axe, Food Is Medicine.* Accessed May 16, 2017. https://draxe.com/lemon-essential-oil-uses-benefits/.

"Top 10 Tea Tree Oil Uses and Benefits." *Dr. Axe, Food Is Medicine.* Accessed May 7, 2017. https://draxe.com/tea-tree-oil-uses-benefits/.

"Top 25 Peppermint Oil Uses and Benefits." *Dr. Axe, Food Is Medicine.* Accessed August 6, 2017. https://draxe.com/peppermint-oil-uses-benefits/.

Traditional Cooking School by GNOWFGLINS. Accessed May 22, 2017.https://traditionalcookingschool.com/?_ga=2.261911629.1196205385.1511812459-486623856.1511812459.

"12 Amazing Neroli Essential Oil Uses." *Dr. Axe, Food Is Medicine.* Accessed May 23, 2017. https://draxe.com/neroli-essential-oil/.

"12 Turmeric Benefits: Superior to Medications?" *Dr. Axe, Food Is Medicine.* Accessed May 7, 2017.https://draxe.com/turmeric-benefits/.

"20 Secret Ways to Use Coconut Oil for Skin." *Dr. Axe, Food Is Medicine.* Accessed July 16, 2017. https://draxe.com/coconut-oil-for-skin/.

"User Guides." *Elizabeth VanBuren.com.* Accessed August 6, 2017. https://elizabethvanburen.com/learn/user-guides/.

"What Is Frankincense Good For? 8 Essential Oil Uses." *Dr. Axe, Food Is Medicine.* Accessed July 9, 2017. https://draxe.com/what-is-frankincense/.

"What Therapeutic Grade Means." *Essential Oils Us.* Accessed May 14, 2017.https://www.essentialoilsus.com/what-therapeutic-grade-mean/.

"Xenoestrogens: 12 Ways to Avoid Them and 24 Ways to Spot Them." *Rachael Pontillo.* Accessed May 9, 2017. https://rachaelpontillo.com/xenoestrogens-12-ways-avoid-24-ways-spot/.

"Xenoestrogens: What Are They, How to Avoid Them." *Women in Balance Institute.* Accessed May 16, 2017. https://womeninbalance.org/2012/10/26/xenoestrogens-what-are-they-how-to-avoid-them/

"Ylang Ylang Boosts Heart Health, Moods & Energy." *Dr. Axe, Food Is Medicine.* Accessed July 9, 2017. https://draxe.com/ylang-ylang/.

"Young Living Essential Oils." Young Living Essential Oils|World Leader in Therapeutic-Grade Essential Oils. Accessed April 27, 2017. https://www.youngliving.com/.

BOOKS

Althea Press: *Essential Oils Natural Remedies: The Complete A–Z.* Berkley, Calif.: 2015.

Lawless, Julia. *The Encyclopedia of Essential Oils: The Complete Guide to the Use of Aromatic Oils in Aromatherapy, Herbalism, Health & Well-Being.* San Francisco: HarperCollins Publishers Ltd., 2002.

Schnaubelt, Kurt. *The Healing Intelligence of Essential Oils.* Rochester, Vermont: Healing Arts Press, 2011.

INDEX

ABOUT THE AUTHOR

AMY LEIGH MERCREE'S motto is "Live joy. Be kind. Love unconditionally." She counsels women and men in the underrated art of self-love to create happier lives. Amy is a bestselling author, media personality, and medical intuitive. Mercree speaks internationally focusing on compassion, joy, and wellness.

Mercree is a bestselling author of eight books including: *The Spiritual Girl's Guide to Dating: Your Enlightened Path to Love, Sex, and Soul Mates, A Little Bit of Chakas: An Introduction to Energy Healing, Joyful Living: 101 Ways to Transform Your Spirit and Revitalize Your Life, The Chakras and Crystals Cookbook: Juices, Sorbets, Smoothies, Salads, and Crystal Infusions to Empower Your Energy Centers, The Compassion Revolution: 30 Days of Living from the Heart, A Little Bit of Meditation,* and *Apple Cider Vinegar Handbook.* Mercree has been featured in *Glamour Magazine, Women's Health, Inc. Magazine, Shape, The Huffington Post, Your Tango, Soul and Spirit Magazine, Mind Body Green,* NBC, CBS, and many more.

Check out AmyLeighMercree.com for articles, picture quotes, and quizzes. Mercree is fast becoming one of the most quoted women on the web. See what all the buzz is about @AmyLeighMercree on Twitter, Snapchat, and Instagram.

✳

To download your FREE essential oils and apple cider vinegar tool kit and power up your health and vitality right now, go to www.amyleighmercree.com/oilandvinegartoolkit—password OILandVINEGAR.